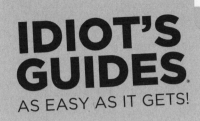

IDIOT'S GUIDES.
AS EASY AS IT GETS!

Ayurveda

by Sahara Rose Ketabi

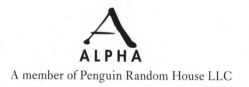

ALPHA

A member of Penguin Random House LLC

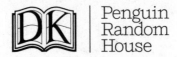

Publisher: Mike Sanders
Associate Publisher: Billy Fields
Acquisitions Editor: Janette Lynn
Cover Designer: Lindsay Dobbs
Book Designer: William Thomas
Compositor: Ayanna Lacey
Proofreader: Lisa Starnes
Indexer: Brad Herriman

First American Edition, 2017
Published in the United States by DK Publishing
6081 E. 82nd Street, Indianapolis, Indiana 46250

ISBN: 9781465462763
Library of Congress Catalog Card Number: 2017930736

Printed and bound in USA

Contents

7   Nature Versus Imbalance 85

8   Lifestyle Practices for Each Dosha.......................... 95

Foreword

In 1991, I wrote *Perfect Health,* the first book to bring Ayurveda to a mainstream Western audience. I felt like a pioneer who couldn't be sure that anyone would follow me. Now, decades later, I've witnessed how Ayurveda steadily rose in popularity until it became almost a household word, certainly among anyone interested in Traditional and integrative medicine. Ayurveda's success is owed, I think, to an urgent need. As our healthcare system became alarmingly expensive, as patients felt frustrated by medical care relying almost entirely on drugs and surgery, the search for alternatives was unstoppable.

Ayurveda has come to the forefront because it is genuinely holistic. It represents not just a traditional approach to healing. A complete analysis of body type, psychological tendencies, specific kinds of imbalances, and dietary requirements opens up a host of lifestyle choices. The benefits have spread far beyond the original conception of the ancient rishis who conceived the principles of Ayurveda. This is a system for lifelong well-being based on the timeless notion that the human body, mind, and spirit are attuned to Nature. When this attunement is maintained through conscious choices in everyday life, the healing response of the body-mind itself is reinforced.

Modern life has reached a level of speed, stress, mechanization, and complexity that the simplicity of remaining in tune with Nature has been forgotten or neglected. Fortunately, we are collectively relearning the basics of wellness. For anyone willing to look deeply enough, this involves a reawakening that begins with questions people have asked for centuries: Who am I? What is this body I inhabit? How do I relate to the vast realm of Nature? Ayurveda provides a totally thought-out, practical approach to these questions. In the West there's a long tradition for connecting Nature and human nature, but nothing as profound and systematic as Ayurveda.

Ayurveda may be the world's oldest health system, but it is in no way dead. In an age where life accelerates too fast, Ayurveda teaches the benefits of going slow by discovering your own natural biorhythms and respecting them. Everyone wants to be healthy—this goes without saying. But as life expectancy has lengthened, the average person in old age spends 8 to 10 years coping with disease and disability. This problem can only be overcome by a long-range strategy for wellness. *Idiot's Guides: Ayurveda* is aimed, therefore, at a mass audience of newcomers who desperately need such a strategy.

This is Ayurveda's next evolutionary step. Sahara Rose has successfully refreshed and revitalized the ancient knowledge without watering down its significance and depth. She blends reverence for the tradition with an awareness of present-day needs. Above all, her book affirms that health surpasses the physical, an idea that ultimately has metaphysical implications when we ponder our place in the universe. Ayurveda views human existence as a mirror of the cosmos. At the very least this connection serves to make us stewards of Earth's ecology, because the planet is our extended body in every process that keeps us alive.

Idiot's Guides: Ayurveda covers a great deal of ground and calls the reader to come back time and time again. Sahara condenses scientific research and spiritual wisdom in a way that suits a time-challenged and information-inundated audience. I believe Sahara will emerge as a leading voice speaking to the millennial generation, who are primed for this paradigm shift. The ideal reader for this book will be inspired, not simply to become part of the Ayurveda movement but to evolve into their own limitless potential.

-Deepak Chopra

World-renowned pioneer in integrative medicine and personal transformation and author of more than 85 books, including numerous *New York Times* best-sellers. Founder of The Chopra Foundation, cofounder of Jiyo.com, and the Chopra Center for Wellbeing.

Introduction

Ayurveda (pronounced *aye-your-VAY-duh*) is the world's oldest health system, stemming from ancient India more than 5,000 years ago. In fact, it's the health system from which all others originated—Chinese, Western, and Herbology included. The Sanskrit word *Ayurveda* means "knowledge of life," and in order to achieve complete health, you must have knowledge of all aspects of your life. This healing system transcends the physical and combines the medical, emotional, mental, spiritual, and metaphysical, which are all interconnected.

Ayurveda dives into the complex mind-body relationship and brings you back into balance—kind of like that blissful feeling you get after a yoga class when you're lying in *shabasana,* or corpse pose. Yes, you can feel like that all the time, and I'm going to teach you how. In this book, I explain not only what Ayurveda is, but also how to apply it easily to your life to transform your health and happiness.

My name is Sahara Rose Ketabi, and I'll be your guide in this sacred journey. I'm a Certified Ayurvedic Pracitioner, Holistic and Sports Nutritionist and wellness blogger behind EatFeelFresh.com I discovered Ayurveda when I needed it most. I was suffering from chronic digestive issues and jumping from one diet to another, searching for the answer to my health. I looked in green smoothies and Paleo forums and finally realized that the answers already existed inside of me, where I never thought to look.

Ayurveda provided me with the tools I needed to tap into the innate wisdom my body already contained. It showed me that the foods that work for me might not work for my friend, family member, or even myself a few months ago. We are constantly changing beings, and our diets and lifestyles need to change, too. A healthy digestion is the secret to a healthy mind, and as soon as I healed my gut, my entire world opened. After that, I vowed to share the tips I learned along the way, from India to Bali to Los Angeles, and now to you.

I wrote this book as the very tool I wish I had when I was lost and confused, trying to figure out what would work for my body. After visiting an Ayurvedic practitioner who knew just about everything going on with me, physically and mentally, I knew Ayurveda's personalized approach to health was what I'd been missing. However, I shied away from Ayurvedic books because I found them confusing and unrelatable, especially with my busy lifestyle and mostly raw vegan diet. I didn't have hours a day to hand-crush exotic Indian herbs, simmer lentils, and perform oil massage. However, I so badly wanted to implement Ayurveda's sacred knowledge into my life because I knew the healing potential it had. This book is simple yet all-encompassing.

I've made the multifaceted healing system of Ayurveda understandable and digestible so you can begin applying it to your life today. I teach you how to master the basics first and then slowly integrate more Ayurvedic practices into your life. I believe true health comes with gradual shifts, not radical decisions that bounce back just as quickly as they come, and my approach provides the framework you need for lifelong balance.

This book is not a set of rules and regulations by which to run your life. It is not a diet, fad, or new theory that will be irrelevant by the time you're done reading it. It's an age-old healing science that has withstood the test of time, and we are returning to it for its tried-and-trued wisdom. I don't expect you to read this book cover to cover in one sitting, but I want it to become your guide, something you refer to for the rest of your life whenever you need it. It's something you can come to when your digestion feels off, you need a spiritual reminder, or you just want to learn more about your body.

I believe the secret to health is merging intuitive ancient wisdom with fact-based modern science because they often point to the same thing, the mind-body connection. Throughout these pages, I offer science-backed research that reaffirms Ayurveda's 5,000-year-old claims, illustrating how the truth is eternal.

Are you ready to empower yourself to become your own healer and finally find the answers you seek inside yourself? Then I invite you to come with me on this journey to discover the ancient healing science of Ayurveda and begin applying it to your life today for radiant, lasting health.

How This Book Is Organized

This book is divided into six parts:

In **Part 1, Ancient Wisdom, Modern Application,** I introduce you to the medical and spiritual system of Ayurveda. I discuss its deep history, why it's regaining popularity, and how it compares to Western medicine and yoga. I also share ways you may already be practicing Ayurveda unknowingly, showing you that the guru is already inside you!

Part 2, Your Unique Mind-Body Type, covers everyone's favorite part of Ayurveda: discovering your *Dosha,* or mind-body type. I give you a quiz to discover your Dosha and share the physical and mental characteristics of each in simple terminology that will finally make sense. I then show you how the Dosha you have today might be different from the one you were born with—and how that's where your imbalances come from. Finally, I offer dietary, lifestyle, and even yoga and meditation advice for your unique Doshic constitution.

Part 3, Establishing an Everyday Routine, is all about lifestyle. I teach you how to set up a daily schedule, including a morning and nighttime routine, for optimal energy, digestion, creativity, sleep, and mind-body balance. I cover everything from oil pulling to tongue scraping to dry brushing, so get ready for some serious self-care in these chapters.

In **Part 4, Ayurvedic Nutrition,** we turn to food. As a Certified Ayurvedic, Holistic, and Sports Nutritionist, this part is really my forte, and I share all the information you need to make it yours, too. I discuss the digestive fire, the Ayurvedic diet philosophy, common nutritional disorders, and toxins in food. In addition, and this is my favorite part, I give you plenty of delicious recipes so you can begin applying this wisdom at tonight's dinner.

Part 5, The Spiritual Side of Ayurveda, contains some of the most important takeaways in the book. What brings many to Ayurveda are the physical benefits, but what makes many stay are the spiritual. This part discusses the three cosmic forces, universal qualities, and energies we are all made of. You may be familiar with your physical body, but I show you that you actually have four more. I also discuss chakras, koshas, and everything in between, bringing you back into your true state: bliss.

In **Part 6, Ayurvedic Healing,** you learn how to apply this ancient healing wisdom in your life. I provide home remedies for everything from digestive disorders to skin conditions to everyday illnesses, teaching you how to become your very own healer.

Extras

Throughout each chapter in this book, you'll find three types of sidebars that hold extra nuggets of wisdom. Here's what to look for:

DEFINITION

Sanskrit can be confusing, but it shouldn't keep you from learning about Ayurveda. In these sidebars, I break down the definitions of complex terminology to help you make sense of it all.

WISDOM OF THE AGES

These sidebars contain insight, useful tips, or just fascinating wisdom that will inspire you.

AYURVEDIC ALERT

Watch out! These sidebars offer cautions of things to be mindful of on your path to achieving mind-body balance with Ayurveda.

Acknowledgments

I first would like to thank the universe for always working in my favor, my spirit guides for leading me in the right direction to fulfill my dharma, my heart for reminding me to always follow my path, my body for housing this human experience, and my soul for filling me with wisdom that sometimes I'm not even sure comes from myself.

In the physical realm, I would like to thank Deepak Chopra for generously writing the foreword to this book, inspiring me more than any other thinker has and believing in me to spread the message of Ayurveda. You have shown me that I am indeed the universe. I would like to thank my parents, Afarin and Mahmoud, for their lifelong support and the many lessons they have taught me along the way—to be strong in my beliefs and wise in my approach; my boyfriend, Steven, for being the Shiva to my Shakti and empowering me with loving care; my brother, Amir, for being my lifelong companion and debate partner; my literary agent, Marilyn Allen, for believing in my vision and allowing it to come to life and into bookstores; my Eat Feel Fresh "Freshie" community, for their years of support on this crazy journey called life; and my readers, for being so receptive to this new yet ancient way of being. Finally, to the era of the divine feminine, I am so honored to be a part of the shift. *Atma Namaste.*

Ancient Wisdom, Modern Application

In Part 1, I introduce you to the medical and spiritual system of Ayurveda. I explain its deep history, look at why it's regaining popularity after being around for more than 5,000 years, and explore how it compares to Western medicine and yoga. I also share ways you may already be practicing Ayurveda without knowing it, showing you that the guru is already inside you!

Discovering Ayurveda

Around 5,000 years ago, Indian sages began developing an intricate system of health and well-being. Through observation and practice, they discovered many secrets to lasting health based on an understanding of an individual's many facets. They orally passed along that wisdom for generations, and eventually it became the leading medical system in India. During the British rule, that system went underground but was still practiced in private homes. After time, that wisdom reemerged and spread far past the borders of India and into the lives of people worldwide as practitioners were drawn to Ayurveda's tried-and-trued methods that have surpassed the test of time.

The lesser-known sister science of yoga, Ayurveda is based on the belief that health can be achieved only through a delicate balance among the mind, body, and spirit. We are all a reflection of our environments and can transform our personal health only through awareness.

In this book, I share this ancient Ayurvedic wisdom with you. Some of these concepts may be totally foreign, while others you may have known your entire life. However, everything will make total sense on an intuitive level because according to Ayurveda, the true secret to health already exists inside you.

In This Chapter

- What Ayurveda is all about
- The lineage of this ancient healing science
- The Ayurveda-yoga connection
- Ayurveda's spiritual and medical practices
- The concept of the digestive fire

What Is Ayurveda?

Ayurveda is a medical science deeply focused on healing and maintaining the quality and longevity of life. Ayurveda combines science with psychology, spirituality, and philosophy, seeing each individual as a microcosm of the universe, with the complexity of the cosmos.

According to Ayurveda, the cornerstone of health is achieving mind-body balance. However, this isn't as simple as it sounds. Ayurveda offers specific guidelines, practices, recipes, and remedies to enable you to achieve this balance. On top of that, the guidelines vary for each person and even change throughout the year, across the seasons, and throughout your lifespan. It sounds complicated, but it is life-changing wisdom that is definitely worth knowing for lifelong well-being.

The Meaning of Ayurveda

Ayurveda actually originates from two separate Sanskrit words: *ayur,* meaning "life," and *veda,* meaning "knowledge." Therefore, to achieve balance, you must have complete knowledge of your life. Ayurveda recognizes that human beings are so much more than physical bodies, rather multidimensional beings with layers of emotions and intuition. Although you may not be "spiritual" per se, the foods you eat and the way you lead your life affect you on a spiritual level every day. Ayurveda helps you recognize that interconnectivity.

> **DEFINITION**
>
> **Ayurveda,** pronounced *aye-your-VAY-duh,* is the science of life based on achieving mind-body balance. It encompasses medical, spiritual, psychological, and philosophical components all focused on promoting lifelong wellness.

The History of Ayurveda

Ayurveda was first discovered in the Indus Valley region of India more than 5,000 years ago. It was passed along orally for generations until it was initially recorded in the ancient Indian *Vedas* or "the books of wisdom." The Vedas are considered the oldest written knowledge in human history and were believed to be composed between 1,700 and 1,000 B.C.E., although some say the knowledge and references they contain date back 10,000 years. The Vedas address everything from ways to heal the body to how to become one with the universe. You could definitely say the *Rishis,* the spiritually enlightened prophets who wrote these texts, were centuries ahead of their time.

How did the original sages discover such knowledge? Nobody exactly knows. They were believed to obtain this innate wisdom directly from the universe to help heal, uplift, and empower the people of this earth. This knowledge was passed down for centuries across generations in memorized chants, known as *sutras*. Ayurveda is the sole system in the Vedas with the purpose of maintaining health because our physical bodies are our vehicles for our spiritual experience.

Around 800 B.C.E., the first Ayurvedic medical school was founded by Punarvasu Atrya, which later influenced Charaka, a scholar who lived around 700 B.C.E. and wrote the *Charaka Samhita*, describing 1,500 different plants and identifying 350 of them as valuable medicine. This text is considered the first major text of Ayurveda. About a century later, the *Susruta Samhita* was written, which formed the basis of modern surgery and is still consulted today.

Ayurveda's comprehensive understanding of the human body was far ahead of its time and became an example for surrounding countries. It eventually spread along what is known as the Silk Road, making its way east from India across China and down to Indonesia. By 400 C.E., Ayurvedic texts were translated into Chinese, and by 700 C.E., Chinese scholars came to India to study Ayurveda, which greatly influenced Chinese medicine.

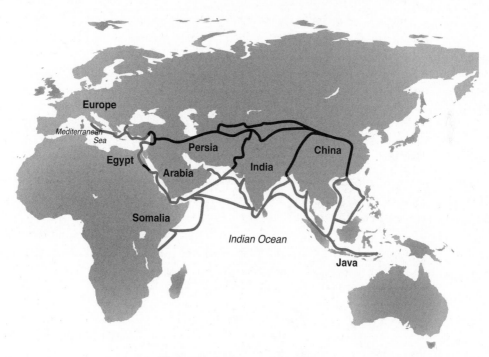

The land and sea routes of the Silk Road.

The science also traveled west across the Persian Empire, up to Europe, farther east to Egypt, and south to Somalia. Arab traders spread the knowledge of Indian herbs in their *Materia Medica*, and this information reached the Greek and Roman Empires, eventually becoming the basis of European medicine and Herbology.

> **WISDOM OF THE AGES**
>
> *Materia medica* is a Latin medical term for the body of collected knowledge about the therapeutic properties of any substance used for healing, inspired by Ayurveda.

The Buddha, born around 550 B.C.E., was a follower of Ayurveda, and the spread of Buddhism across Asia was accompanied by the practice of Ayurveda. In a period when so little was known about the human mind and body, Ayurveda explained the cause of diseases; the symptoms of imbalance; the unique body types; and ways to achieve mental, emotional, and spiritual well-being.

Unfortunately, during the British rule over India, Ayurveda was considered an archaic practice and no longer permitted. Western medicine was forced upon the Indian people, who privately refused to let go of the traditions in their own homes. Ayurveda went underground and lived on through home remedies and recipes that are finally regaining popularity today. Ayurveda became a "kitchen medicine" that healed families with food, spices, oils, and herbs. The city of Kerala in southern India became a safe haven for Ayurveda, and today, it boasts many Ayurvedic centers and institutions. Currently, Ayurveda is experiencing a renaissance, as people struggling with Western medicine crave a more holistic approach to their physical and mental well-being and turn to this ancient wisdom.

Ayurveda Today

Ayurveda is practiced not only in the India subcontinent but also globally. Oil pulling, dry brushing, and self-oil massage are now hitting the mainstream. Much of the wisdom we know about food combining and digestion derives from Ayurvedic knowledge. Turmeric, now being sold in capsules for its antinflammatory, antioxidant, antidepressant and anti-aging benefits, has always been a staple spice in the Ayurvedic diet. Thousands of people travel to India each year to partake in Ayurvedic *Panchakarma* treatments to detoxify and rejuvenate their health. What's more, Ayurveda is practiced by millions of people every day who may not even know they are practicing it.

> 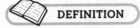 **DEFINITION**
>
> **Panchakarma** is a fivefold detoxification and rejuvenation treatment in Ayurveda, involving massage, herbal therapy, and other treatments.

People today are sick and tired of the one-size-fits-all approach to health that has left Americans in a less-than-optimal state of health. They are drawn to Ayurveda's whole-body approach to health that sees the entire person, rather than just a single symptom. In a time when doctors rarely have time to get to know the individual, people are left on their own to determine the root cause of their diseases. Ayurveda can help unravel those mysteries.

According to Ayurveda, health does not come in the form of a pill or prescription, but rather in a balanced lifestyle. Although a balanced lifestyle regiment is a lot more difficult to follow than taking a prescription, and requires personal responsibility to maintain, it's far more effective.

One of the tenets of Ayurveda is that the secret of well-being depends on the unique individual. We all have distinctive genetic makeups, lifestyles, physiologies, metabolisms, mental characteristics, and a host of other factors that determine our medical and dietary needs. This concept of individuality hits home with people who have grown weary of general health statements that have left them feeling depleted and defeated.

According to Ayurveda, no single guideline can work for all people because we are all different beings with unique needs. Although this may seem like an obvious finding, it actually took several thousands of years, an obesity epidemic, and a health crisis for many of us to figure out. Ayurveda really was far ahead of its time.

Ayurvedic Versus Western Medicine

Ayurvedic medicine is not meant to replace Western medicine but rather to complement it. Its focus is more preventative, whereas conventional medicine's concentration is more symptomatic. Ayurveda's approach to health is to inhibit the disease from appearing. The Western approach to health is to deal with the disease after it has appeared. Today, Western medicine is highly advanced in treating acute conditions and trauma due to its technical sophistication. However, it lacks the understanding of the interconnectivity of these symptoms and the reasons why they keep reoccurring, which Ayurveda uncovers.

Ayurvedic medicine upholds that our physical conditions reflect our mental and vice versa. If a person is experiencing liver issues, an Ayurvedic practitioner will ask them about their unresolved anger. If a person is overweight, they will ask them what they may be emotionally holding on to. If someone is unable to sleep, they will recommend they ground themselves by walking in nature. An Ayurvedic practitioner won't provide suggestions until they know about your childhood, your eating patterns, your daily schedule, and even your dreams. They do not look just at a problem, but rather at all of the factors that may have caused it. They offer a holistic approach, including the whole person—body, mind, and spirit.

Ayurvedic medicine does include surgeries, medical examinations, and other procedures, which I discuss later in this chapter, but today, those procedures are less practiced than Ayurveda's everyday dietary and lifestyle recommendations. Many Ayurvedic herbs are available—some being pure and highly effective, others less so. As with any medicine, it's important to know what you're putting in your body rather than taking something just because it says it's Ayurvedic. However, the best and most effective medicine you can consume is the food on your plate.

WISDOM OF THE AGES

The best Ayurvedic herbs are organic, obtained straight from a reliable source, and recommended by a professional.

Ayurveda and Yoga

Today, 30 percent of Americans have practiced yoga, and that number is on the rise. The increasingly widespread practice of yoga has made more people interested in Ayurveda, its sister practice. The Vedas intended these sciences to be practiced together, although Ayurveda is only now beginning to get some of its more popular sister's spotlight.

If you've taken a yoga class, what was your reasoning behind your practice? Was it to become one with a divine source, or was it to become healthier and more balanced? If the former, then you were truly practicing yoga. If the latter, then you were actually practicing Ayurveda.

Ayurveda's purpose is to achieve health, while yoga's is to achieve spiritual enlightenment. In fact, most people at yoga classes are likely practicing Ayurveda, rather than yoga, because it's the health benefits they seek rather than oneness with the divine.

WISDOM OF THE AGES

Ayurveda and yoga go hand in hand because we cannot become our *highest* selves if we are not our *healthiest* selves. Our bodies are temporary vessels holding our eternal souls. They were given to us to experience this amazing gift called life. It's up to us to treat them with profound love and care.

The better we nourish our bodies, the more in tune with our inner consciousness we become. This is why yoga is a recommended practice in Ayurveda, and Ayurveda is a recommended practice in yoga. The healthier we become, the more spiritually aware we become. The daily practices in Ayurveda have a purpose, and that is to elevate our consciousness. Health is not the end goal but rather the means for it. The end goal is awakening and transcendence. Self-awareness, scientific knowledge, *asanas* (yoga poses), meditation, and healing modalities are only tools to help us get there.

A Spiritual and Medical System

When most of us think of medicine and spirituality, we think of two opposite ends of a spectrum. However, Ayurveda blends these two disciplines harmoniously. It merges our left and right brains into one multifaceted system that includes all aspects of a human being.

According to Ayurveda, even before they manifest, we can feel illnesses by the subtle layers of our energetic body, which I address further in Chapter 20. If you've ever had a sense that something was "off" before it turned into a sickness, that was your subtle energy calling. Ayurveda marries the seen and unseen to create a comprehensive discipline of spiritual and medical well-being.

Ayurveda's Two Main Principles

Ayurveda teaches two main principles:

Preservation of health: How to maintain wellness and what to do to keep your body healthy and fit to avoid illness.

Methods, medicine, and tactics for disease management and ailments: How to cure and procure a return to health.

The first principle is based on prevention, while the second is based on regaining balance. The two are important and meant to be practiced together.

The Eight Branches of Ayurveda

Ayurvedic science consists of eight branches, collectively called *Ashtang Ayurveda*. The word *ashtang* means "eight," and you'll see the number 8 pop up in various areas of the Vedas. Yoga similarly has eight branches.

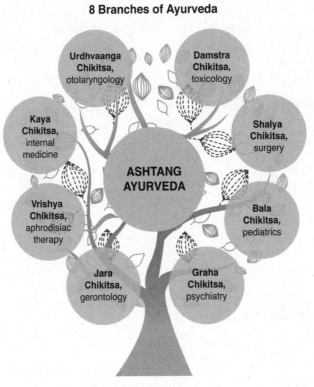

The eight branches of Ayurveda.

Let's take a look at the eight branches:

Kaya Chikitsa, **also known as internal medicine:** This psychosomatic practice states that the mind can create disease in the body and vice versa. Its purpose is finding the root cause of an illness and its connection to the mind, body, and soul. This theory describes the three Doshas: *Vata, Pitta,* and *Kapha,* which I discuss further in Chapters 3 and 4. Ayurvedic herbal treatments, detoxification, diets, and healing therapies are all part of Kaya Chikitsa and the main focuses of this book.

Urdhvaanga Chikitsa, **commonly known as otolaryngology:** This portion of Ayurvedic medicine is solely related to the head and neck. Ayurveda lists 72 eye diseases and surgical procedures for many eye-related disorders, including cataracts and eyelid diseases. It also contains surgeries and treatments for the ears, nose, and throat.

Damstra Chikitsa, **which refers to toxicology:** According to Ayurveda, the air we breathe is as important as the food we eat, the environment in which we live, and the thoughts we think. Damstra Chikitsa is focused on toxicology and addresses air and water pollution; toxins in animals, minerals, and vegetables; and health epidemics.

Shalya Chikitsa, **which is surgery:** Ayurveda's sophisticated surgical methods influenced the ancient Egyptian, Greek, Roman, Persian, and Chinese empires. Common surgeries included bladder stone and intestinal obstruction removal.

Bala Chikitsa, **also called pediatrics:** This part of Ayurveda includes pre- and postnatal care of mother and baby as well as childhood health.

Graha Chikitsa, **which signifies psychiatry:** Ayurveda finds mental well-being an extremely important facet of health. This branch incorporates meditation, yoga, and breathing techniques to overcome anxiety, depression, anger, and other imbalances.

Jara Chikitsa, **also called gerontology:** This refers to the scientific study of old age, the process of aging, and particular problems of the elderly. It also addresses longevity and practices you can do, such as fasting, to promote longer lifespans.

Vrishya Chikitsa, **which relates to aphrodisiac therapy:** Sexual health is an important component of Ayurveda because it sustains life. Intimacy can promote spiritual evolvement and strengthen partnerships. Vrishya Chikitsa deals both with fertility-related issues as well as the treatment of sexual dysfunctions.

As you can see, Ayurveda is an integrative system of health that covers many aspects of healing. It overlaps with many fields of Western medicine and also covers some entirely distinct areas of study.

The Secret to Health

According to Ayurveda, the secret to health lies in the digestive system. The Ayurvedic word for digestion is the Sanskrit term for fire, *agni*. Our digestion is our eternal fire, powering us through life. This digestive fire is responsible for all transformation in the body, including the metabolism, nutrient absorption, and elimination. I share more about this internal fire in Chapter 12.

Not only do you digest food, but you also digest emotions, senses, and experiences. If your agni is not burning bright, you feel stuck and depleted, both physically and mentally. Unprocessed emotions are just as harmful as unprocessed foods, adding heaviness and toxicity to the mind and body.

AYURVEDIC ALERT

Unresolved emotions can cause mental and physical imbalances in your body, including weight gain and stress-related disorders. It's important to work through your past for a brighter future.

Many mental imbalances you feel are related to our digestive issues. Depression is caused by a slow, weak digestive fire, making you feel stuck and depleted. An overly active digestive fire causes irritability and impatience. Anxiety and restlessness may be caused by too much gas accumulation in the system. Each of these imbalances is related to your unique Dosha.

The Ayurvedic View of Health

The Ayurvedic view of health is to have a body without pain or illness so you are free to evolve spiritually. When you are sick, you are unable to even think about anything besides getting better. You become stuck in your physical body and obsessed with finding a way to regain health. However, when you're healthy, you're no longer concerned with your physical body. You surpass the physical and reach *self-actualization,* which is the realization or fulfillment of one's talents and potentialities.

> **DEFINITION**
>
> **Self-actualization** is the achievement of one's full potential through creativity, independence, spontaneity, and a grasp of the real world.

To achieve health, you must be physically, emotionally, spiritually, occupationally, and environmentally sound. If any of these components is missing, you won't truly feel health. For example, if you have a strong body and a great job but weak relationships, the rest of you will suffer. Your emotional imbalance will become a spiritual imbalance that will eventually manifest into physical ailments, which will affect your occupation and those around you. All aspects of your health are interconnected, and if you aren't balanced in all areas, your entire being suffers.

The Ayurvedic View of Life

According to Vedic philosophy, human life has a definitive purpose, which is split into four pursuits: *dharma, artha, kama,* and *moksha.*

Dharma is the comprehensive term for the 10 values every person should have. These principles are as follows:

Wisdom: You must always try to become wiser through study, personal experience, and learning from others.

Truth: You must always be true in thought, words, and actions.

Forbearance: You must remain calm and composed in all circumstances.

Control of senses: You must control your senses and learn to master your emotions.

Control of mind: You must exercise full control over your mind, which is always restless.

Forgiveness: You must forgive others, for it makes you physically and morally stronger. However, it isn't advisable to forgive someone who has done you wrong multiple times.

Nonstealing: You must never steal or take something from another without asking permission.

Cleanliness: You must keep your body, home, and mind clear and pure.

Nonanger: You must resist anger, even when provoked.

Knowledge: You must always seek knowledge of the physical and spiritual domains from all possible sources.

Artha is the acquisition of wealth. This doesn't refer to only material wealth, but rather the four forms of artha:

Knowledge: Knowledge is the greatest form of wealth. It transcends material wealth because spiritual knowledge cannot be lost and leads to true fulfillment.

Health: Health includes physical, emotional, mental, and spiritual well-being. Good food, exercise, and thoughts are required for proper health.

Contentment: Contentment means being happy with what you have and letting go of the need to possess and become more. Contentment is a form of wealth because it provides mental peace and moral strength.

Material wealth: It's important to be able to financially sustain yourself and not depend on others for your needs. Money is energy, and you should value your time and expertise. You should not become a slave of material wealth, but learn to master it.

Kama is the controlled fulfillment of desires. It contains two facets:

- You must have desires in life because that's what inspire you to discover and give back.

- You must not be controlled by your desires because that leads to destruction.

 AYURVEDIC ALERT

Be mindful of your desires! You should have desires without being attached to their outcome. Your desires must be kept in check to make your life useful and purposeful without becoming deluded by wanting more.

Moksha is the fourth and final objective to human life and is the ultimate goal of existence. This is the state of *Ananda*—pure bliss—which, once you've attained it, you desire nothing more. It's the wealth of pure liberation. You are no longer driven by your desires but can relax into your being. This is the highest objective of life and can only be achieved once you have attained the first three objectives, dharma, artha, and kama. You must start small to become infinite.

Digesting Food and Thoughts: Ojas and Ama

Ayurveda focuses on health to achieve transcendence. By cleaning up your diet, you clean up your life. You create space for positivity and detach yourself from the things that have been holding you back. You build *ojas,* which is the Ayurvedic term for "vigor" and "the physiological expression of consciousness." Ojas results from clear digestion. When you are able to break down your food, assimilate nutrients, and evacuate them from your body effectively, you feel radiant, refreshed, and rejuvenated.

However, when food sits in your gastrointestinal tract for too long, toxins accumulate, which are called *ama.* Ama is the underlying cause of nearly every health issue. A healthy, pure body does not suddenly become ill. It becomes ill as the result of built-up toxicity, year after year, that isn't eliminated from the body.

Ojas is the life force; ama is toxicity. You have both in your body, and with a balanced diet and lifestyle, you can eliminate ama and radiate with ojas.

Let's take a moment to assess where you stand. Don't worry about not quite being a pinnacle of perfect health yet; you've just started your journey and now is the perfect time to start. The following table outlines symptoms of ojas and ama so you can determine which is more prevalent in you today.

Signs of Ojas	Signs of Ama
You wake up feeling rested.	You wake up exhausted.
Your tongue is clear and pink.	Your tongue has a white coating.
You have a clear, glowing complexion.	You suffer from acne, blemishes, or other skin problems.
You feel steadily energized throughout the day.	You have an energy crash midday and often need sugar, caffeine, or a nap.
You enjoy eating abundant vegetables and don't have food cravings.	You don't like the taste of vegetables and often crave foods.
You can digest food easily without feeling bloated, gassy, or tired.	You often feel bloated, gassy, or tired after meals.
Your body has a pleasant smell.	Your sweat tends to have a sharp, foul odor.
Your mind is clear and peaceful.	You constantly get anxious, angry, or depressed.
You rarely become ill.	You are susceptible to infections.
You can fall asleep soundly.	You have difficulty falling sleep.

Where do you stand? You can be honest with yourself; no one is judging. If you're more on the ama side, have no fear. That will change by the time you're through reading—and implementing—the suggestions in this book.

Beginning Your Journey

Now you know what Ayurveda is all about and how it connects with all facets of your life. Perhaps you've never heard of Ayurveda before this book and these concepts are totally new to you. Perhaps you've been practicing yoga for many years and want to take a deeper look at its roots. Regardless of your background, this book came to you for a reason.

There are no coincidences in life. Ayurveda's ancient wisdom was put in your hands to transform your life. In this book, I help you achieve mind-body balance, heal those around you, and actualize your potential through the practices of Ayurveda. I know how overwhelming Ayurveda can be so I simplify this complex science without watering it down, using terminology you can understand and relate to. I provide the practices, recipes, and remedies you need to bring this ancient wisdom off the pages of this book and into your life. All I ask is that you listen to the voice within.

The Least You Need to Know

- Ayurveda is a comprehensive medical and spiritual system that merges the mind, body, and spirit.
- Ayurveda is the world's oldest health system—at least 5,000 years old—and is still practiced globally.
- Ayurveda is the sister science of yoga with the purpose of health and well-being, while yoga's purpose is spiritual awakening.
- When you are healthy, you are full of ojas—vibrant, energized, balanced, and peaceful. When you are unhealthy, you are full of ama—exhausted, lazy, smelly, and sick.
- The purpose of health surpasses the physical body and instead is achieving self-actualization, which enables you to reach your highest potential.

Practicing Ayurveda

Ayurveda might seem like a totally foreign practice with tons of guidelines the average person could never adhere to, but this couldn't be further from the truth! Ayurveda is a highly intuitive lifestyle that's actually extremely easy to follow. In fact, many of the common health practices performed today are actually Ayurvedic.

In this chapter, I explain what practicing Ayurveda is all about, from eating seasonally to meditation. Then, I bust some common myths and show you how easy it is to bring more Ayurvedic wisdom into your life—if it isn't in there already!

In This Chapter

- Are you already (unknowingly) practicing Ayurveda?
- Ayurvedic rituals such as oil pulling and dry brushing
- Common misconceptions about Ayurveda
- Easy ways to implement Ayurvedic practices in your lifestyle

You May Be Practicing Ayurveda Already

Do you use oils in your diet or beauty regimen? Switch up your diet from summer to fall? Practice yoga or meditation? Take herbs to heal common ailments or drink herbal tea? Use a brush to exfoliate your skin? Scrape your tongue? If you do any of these, you are practicing Ayurveda already.

One of the greatest things about Ayurveda is its simplicity. It doesn't require expensive super-foods, fancy kitchen appliances, or a strict diet regimen. Ayurveda was created thousands of years ago, before these things even existed. The founders of Ayurveda discovered healing uses of the things around them, from common herbs to oils. Food was seen as medicine, and each meal was your daily prescription.

Because Ayurveda was the first health system, much of what we practice today actually stems from Ayurvedic tradition. The way we think about food, beauty, and medicine comes from Ayurvedic influences. Today more than ever before, people are looking back at this ancient wisdom for its long-standing existence. If you are a coconut oil addict, home remedy maven, or herbal tea connoisseur, you are practicing Ayurveda already.

Your Morning Routine

We all have some sort of morning routine we follow to get ready for the day. Yours might include brushing your teeth while running to the toaster to heat up a couple slices of bread before getting your kids ready for school. Or maybe it's hitting the snooze button five times until you drag yourself out of bed and somehow make it to work by the time you wake up, coffee in hand. Perhaps you jump out of bed, chug a big bottle of water, put on your sneakers, and push your body through an hour-long workout followed by a cold shower and icy protein shake. Maybe you're one who naturally wakes up when the sun rises, slowly allows your body to get ready for the day, warm tea in hand, while either journaling or lightly stretching. Is one routine better than the others? I'll let you decide when you're done reading this book.

Whatever your current morning routine, the fact that you have one is a sort of Ayurvedic ritual. In Sanskrit, your daily routine is called your *dinacharya,* or "to be close to the day." This means being in touch with the earth's natural cycles, such as waking up when the sun rises and going to sleep when it sets. However, it gets much deeper than that, which I discuss more in Chapters 9 and 10.

DEFINITION

Dinacharya is your daily practice, such as brushing your teeth, washing your face, scraping your tongue, oiling your body, meditating, and eating breakfast. It is highly recommended to have some sort of routine in Ayurveda.

According to Ayurveda, the way you start your day is how you'll feel for the rest of the day. If you begin your day in a rush, you'll feel nervous and restless for the duration of the day. If you start slow and tired, you'll feel lazy and heavy for the rest of the day. If you overexert yourself at the beginning of the day, you'll feel burnt out for the rest of the day. It's all about maintaining a very fine balance of waking yourself up without wearing yourself out.

Ayurvedic morning practices include the following:

Oil pulling: This is swishing around oil in your mouth to remove toxins, similar to using mouthwash.

Tongue scraping: This is scraping your tongue with a copper scraper to remove toxic buildup, similar to brushing your tongue with your toothbrush.

Abhyanga: This is self-oil massage to stimulate your lymphatic system, similar to applying lotion.

Dry brushing: This is brushing your skin with a dry brush to remove dead skin cells, similar to using a loofa.

These practices aren't totally foreign; you might be doing many of them already. I explain more on how you can incorporate these, and other Ayurvedic practices, into your daily routine in Chapters 10 and 11.

Herbal Teas and Remedies

If you drink herbal tea or take herbal supplements, you are practicing Ayurveda. As more people become aware of the dehydrating effects of caffeine and the potential risks of Western drugs, they are switching to more herbal teas and remedies. Coffee shops around the country now offer a rich selection of herbal teas, such as chamomile or rooibos. Pharmacies similarly boast growing sections of herbal supplements to treat a host of symptoms, from hormonal imbalance to unstable blood sugar levels. People are turning back to nature to cure their imbalances. Ayurveda was the first health system to use herbs for medicinal benefits, and modern Herbology is based on Ayurveda.

Herbal remedies are nothing new to the majority of the world. In fact, the World Health Organization has estimated that 80 percent of the world's population uses traditional therapies, a major part of which are derived from plants. Ayurveda recommends a wide range of herbs, from ginger to triphala, to heal the body from within.

The use of herbal supplements is steadily increasing in the United States. In 2012, one in five Americans was using herbal, nonvitamin supplements, and that number has continued to increase. Americans spent at least $21 billion on herbs and other dietary supplements in 2015. In fact, according to the National Institutes of Health, one third of Americans uses alternative medicine, including herbal supplements, meditation, yoga, and chiropractic adjustments.

Herbal supplements are often an attractive alternative to pharmaceuticals because they offer the same benefits with a decreased risk of side effects. For example, there are no risks of adding too much ginger to your food, besides making it too spicy, because ginger is a root vegetable grown naturally. Our bodies are able to recognize plant-based ingredients, allowing them to cooperate more with our systems.

Herbal treatments also are desirable because they are more affordable than pharmaceutical drugs. For example, the arthritis drug Celebrex costs more than $4 per day, whereas ginger supplements, an Ayurvedic arthritis treatment, cost about 38¢ per day. Even less expensive is adding fresh grated ginger to your meals and teas.

Herbal teas are a large part of the Ayurvedic diet and are actually viewed as medicine. Instead of medicine, as an Ayurvedic practitioner, I often "prescribe" my clients specific tea recipes with certain spices they need to address their underlying issues.

WISDOM OF THE AGES

Teas are an effective way of consuming herbs because their benefits are enhanced when steeped in hot water. Herbal teas are a great alternative to caffeinated black tea or coffee, which dehydrate the body and put the adrenals on overdrive. Ayurveda recommends countless unique tea recipes, some sweet and others quite bitter, depending on what the individual needs. Common teas include ginger, fennel, and peppermint.

Each herbal tea has a multitude of benefits. Whereas pharmaceutical drugs are intended for only one purpose, most herbs have numerous. Ginger tea is not only medicinal for arthritis, but also a powerful aid for improving digestion and reducing inflammation. Fennel tea relieves gas, bloating, and constipation while also detoxifying the liver. Similarly, peppermint tea relieves nausea, vomiting, and stomachaches, while also cooling the body. Specific herbs are recommended for each body type, season, and environment.

Ayurveda recommends making your own herbal teas to reap the benefits in the most natural form, without the potential risk of chemicals in conventional tea bags. Grated ginger, fennel seeds, or peppermint is all you need, which is also much more affordable than buying tea. Most of the teas Ayurveda recommends are used in cooking as well, and you don't need too many staples. For teas where you may not have the original ingredient, you can purchase loose-leaf tea. Loose-leaf tea is preferable to bagged tea to avoid potential toxins and pesticides.

AYURVEDIC ALERT

Ayurveda recommends making your own tea with common spices or buying loose-leaf tea to avoid potential pesticides and chemicals in bagged tea. Always avoid plastic tea bags because the plastic leaches into the hot water. Do your research on the manufacturer, and always opt for organic when buying tea.

Oils

We recently went through a time when people were afraid of oils. We were told that oils in our food would make us fat and should be avoided. Similarly, oils in our skincare products were supposed to cause acne and breakouts.

Today, thankfully, we have learned this isn't true. All fats don't make us fat, and not all oil on our skin causes acne—and some can actually heal it. Those same outlets that once advocated the abandonment of oil now have become oil obsessed. They recommend adding oil to your cooking, putting it on your skin, and making it into masks for your hair—something Ayurveda has advocated about for 5,000 years.

WISDOM OF THE AGES

In Ayurveda, oil is love. In fact, the Sanskrit word for oil, *sneha*, actually means "love." To oil your body is an act of self-love. Abhyanga, self-oil massage, is an integral part of the dinacharya daily practice.

Adding oil to your food makes it easier to digest. The oil allows for the breakdown of the food and enables your gastrointestinal tract to better process the food. Difficult-to-digest foods like fibrous cauliflower and kale should always be paired with oil.

Oil is also the key to hydration. Your cells cannot absorb water without oil. That's why a diet low in oil can leave you dehydrated. Dehydration affects your body inside and out. A lack of oil in your diet causes constipation internally and dry or dull skin, frizzy or split end-prone hair, and cracked lips and nails externally.

The beauty industry has scared many of us away from using oil on our faces because we've been told it clogs pores. That's true for mineral oils found in lotions and makeup as well as animal oils. These oils form a waterproof film on top of the skin's debris, locking in bacteria, dead skin cells, sweat, and sebum.

However, plant-based oils are similar to the kinds our skin produces naturally and are easily absorbed by the skin without clogging pores. They're more moisturizing than creams and lotions because they bind moisture to the skin while strengthening skin cell membranes. Oil can be used both for cleansing the skin as well as moisturizing it, which I explain more in Chapter 11.

Ayurveda recommends specific oils for the individual Doshas, or mind-body types. For those with more dry, rough skin, warming sesame oil is recommended. For acne-prone, oily skin, cooling coconut oil is recommended. For moist, combination skin, sesame, almond, or olive oil is recommended, depending on the season.

> **AYURVEDIC ALERT**
>
> Oils can be used topically or internally because according to Ayurveda, you shouldn't put anything on your skin that you wouldn't also eat. Your skin is your largest organ, and whatever you rub on your body makes its way into your bloodstream. Be sure it's free of parabens, alcohols, fragrances, and chemicals.

More Ayurvedic Practices

Do you brush your skin with a loofa? Turns out, that practice is best outside the shower. Dry brushing, the Ayurvedic practice of scrubbing your body with a dry brush to remove dead skin, is regaining popularity. According to Ayurveda, it's important to exfoliate your skin so your cells can breathe without a rough layer of dead skin smothering them. I explain more about how to dry brush in Chapter 11.

Have you ever used a tongue scraper? That's another Ayurvedic practice hitting the modern mainstream. Ayurveda recommends scraping your tongue with a copper scraper to remove ama, or toxins, that have accumulated overnight. As you sleep, your mouth breeds bacteria from your gut, and it's important to remove them not only for mouth health but also for digestive well-being. I explain more about tongue scraping in Chapter 10.

After a shower, do you ever rub oil in your skin? You guessed it—also Ayurvedic. When practiced the right way, this self-oil massage, or abhyanga, stimulates the lymphatic system, calms the mind and body, and allows your body to release toxins. It can be practiced on your own or professionally in an Ayurvedic massage treatment, part of a *Panchakarma*, which I discuss in Chapter 22.

As mentioned earlier, Ayurveda has many ancient practices that are in use today. Although many Americans probably have never heard the word *Ayurveda*, much of their self-care and dietary routines originate from Ayurvedic traditions. You may be dabbling in some Ayurvedic practices already, and this book teaches you many more. Ayurveda doesn't have to be complicated or time-consuming. In fact, there are many misconceptions about Ayurveda that I debunk next.

Misconceptions About Ayurveda

Some people who have dabbled a bit in Ayurvedic studies may have concluded that it is arduous and archaic or means you have to eat vegetarian curry for the rest of your life. None of these things are true. Ayurveda can be applied to any lifestyle, whether you eat meat, dislike Indian food, or barely have time to cook. In this section, I dispel some common misconceptions about Ayurveda so you can see for yourself how easy it is to follow Ayurvedic guidelines.

Ayurveda Is Time-Consuming

I totally understand this assumption because I made it myself when I was studying Ayurveda in India and thinking how impossible it would be to follow the guidelines when I returned to the United States. However, I since have found it to be completely false. Boiling a pot of beans takes about 1 minute to prepare. Throwing together vegetables and spices in my slow cooker takes about 5. Many of the Ayurvedic recipes I follow are prepared in just one pot. In fact, I have saved time and money by following an Ayurvedic diet because many of the staples, like rice and lentils, are extremely affordable and easy to prepare. All I do is add some herbs and spices, and my meals are ready.

You Have to Be a Vegetarian

Ayurveda does recommend following a mostly vegetarian diet because meat is difficult for the body to digest, but it doesn't mean you have to be vegetarian. In fact, Ayurveda actually recommends the consumption of meat in two scenarios.

The first is if you are extremely weak, such as if you have an autoimmune disease or are malnourished, and need meat to regain strength. In this case, meat is seen as medicine. Eating it is considered honoring the circle of life because you are taking life in order to survive. High-quality meat provides a great deal of sustenance to the body, which is necessary for those with debilitating diseases or malnourished bodies. Patients are encouraged to eat organic and/or grass-fed meat until they regain health and then can revert to a mostly meat-free diet because plant-based foods have all the protein we need.

The second group Ayurveda recommends meat for is the "warrior caste." These were the protectors of the land at the time Ayurveda developed. Meat was recommended for the warriors because it invokes qualities of *rajas,* filling them up with powerful energy and vigor—a desirable trait for those protecting the civilization. We don't have a warrior caste today, but we definitely have people who overexert themselves physically. Those who are extremely active, such as weight lifters and athletes, and need extra protein to rejuvenate their muscles fall in this category. It's not necessary for most people, but an option Ayurveda includes.

The reason Ayurveda does not recommend eating meat regularly is because it's not easy to digest. Our gastrointestinal tracts are far longer than those of carnivorous animals. We also lack the stomach acid lions and tigers have. This causes the meat we consume to sit in our bellies, rotting and causing toxic accumulation, or ama. Ama causes countless imbalances, such as kidney stones, gout, gallstones, ulcers, and other disorders. Many believe a high-protein diet helps them lose weight, but research has shown that consuming excess protein actually has the same effect as consuming excess carbohydrates and causes fat accumulation.

Ayurveda has no strict labels, only fluid suggestions. There may be times in your life when you could benefit from meat, such as if you're overworked, malnourished, overexerted, or fatigued. There may be times when you're better on a completely plant-based diet. Some people may need meat several times a year, while others several times a week. What's important is that you check in with your body to see what you truly need and get out of the habit of eating animal products at every meal just because.

The amount of animal products you might need in your diet changes according to the season and your environment. In the colder, winter months, you need more fats in your diet. Because of the lower temperatures, the saturated fat in meat can help you preserve body heat. You'll notice that in countries with colder climates, more meat is consumed for that reason. In the summer, you need more fresh fruit and vegetables to cool down.

Whether you choose to eat meat or not is entirely your decision. If you do, Ayurveda recommends specific types of animal products for each body type, which I discuss in Chapter 6. It is possible to include meat in your diet while following Ayurvedic guidelines, as long as you consume it when your body truly needs it, pay the animal respect, and are certain it was farmed sustainably.

> **WISDOM OF THE AGES**
>
> Ayurveda is a mostly vegetarian diet that recommends meat in two situations—if you're extremely weak or if you overexert yourself physically. In both cases, meat should be organic and/or grass-fed and respect must be paid to the animal for giving its life for your sustenance.

It Only Includes Indian Food

This is another judgment I made while studying Ayurveda in India because frankly, every recipe I learned was Indian! As much as I love Indian food, it wasn't the only food I wanted to eat for the rest of my life. So I started creating my own recipes, using Ayurvedic guidelines but with ingredients found near me, such as kale, berries, quinoa, and avocados. It is entirely possible to eat Ayurvedically without eating only traditional Indian Ayurvedic foods.

Ayurveda is more of a framework on what to eat and how. You don't have to consume just traditional Ayurvedic recipes to benefit from Ayurvedic wisdom. These recipes were created thousands of years ago, in India, and contain ingredients found only in the region. Instead, you can apply Ayurvedic suggestions, such as food combining, eating for your Dosha, changing your diet according to the season, and noticing the qualities of your food, to any type of food—Italian, Mexican, French, you name it. Ayurveda teaches you how to make that food healthier for your body.

Anybody Can Practice Ayurveda

Ayurveda doesn't require hours of cooking, fancy kitchen equipment, tofu-only dinners, or a lifetime of Indian cuisine. Ayurveda can make its way into your life easily and painlessly, from the way you start your day to the way you prepare your meals. Ayurveda offers many recommendations, and you can pick and choose what works best for you.

There's no need to change 100 percent of your life overnight to strictly follow the Ayurvedic guidelines. The beauty of Ayurveda is that it's a lifelong practice. You have the rest of your existence to adapt a more Ayurvedic lifestyle. Take one thing at a time, and let it become a routine. Once that one thing has become habitual, include something else. Consistency is key and much more effective than a crash diet followed by reverting to fast food and sugar.

Ayurveda has so many gifts to offer. The only question is which you'd like to receive first.

The Least You Need to Know

- Ayurvedic practices aren't so out of reach, and you might be practicing many already.
- The way you start your day is the way you'll feel for the rest of your day, so choose carefully.
- Herbal teas and remedies are an integral part of Ayurveda and best in their most natural form.
- You do not have to be a strict vegetarian to follow Ayurveda; you can eat organic, grass-fed meat only when your body truly needs it.
- Eat seasonally and locally to ensure you are eating the right foods for your body at the right times of the year.

The Cornerstone of Ayurveda

Ayurveda is more than a medical science; it's a multifaceted philosophy based on the earth's natural elements. You are a reflection of your environment, and the fire, wind, and waters of the earth exist within you.

In this chapter, I discuss the cornerstone of Ayurveda, the philosophies it's based on, the elements it relates to, the layers of your body, and the three universal qualities that exist in all things.

In This Chapter

- Exploring the Vedas and Ayurveda's sister sciences, the Upavedas
- Discovering the five elements: fire, earth, water, air, and ether (space)
- Introducing the three Doshas: Vata, Pitta, and Kapha
- What each Dosha governs in the mind and body

The Vedas

Although Ayurveda was passed on orally for many generations, it was first written down in the Vedas, the most ancient Sanskrit text, on which Hinduism is based. The Vedas are books of wisdom that offer guidelines on how to live your life for optimal well-being. (The word *Veda* itself means "knowledge.") There are four main Vedas:

1. The Rig Veda: The Book of Mantra (estimated to be written between 3000 and 2500 B.C.E.) (it needs a "the" in front of it, like the Bible or the Torah)

2. The Yajur Veda: The Book of Ritual (estimated to be written between 1200 and 1000 B.C.E.), Sam Veda (1200 to 1000 B.C.E.), and Atharva Veda (1200 to 1000 B.C.E.)

3. The Sama Veda: The Book of Chant (estimated to be written between 1200 and 1000 B.C.E.)

4. The Atharva Veda: The Book of Magical Formulas (estimated to be written between 1200 and 1000 B.C.E.)

Following these four Vedas are four secondary teachings, called the *Upavedas*. Ayurveda is one of these Upavedas and the sole system in the Vedas with the purpose of improving health.

The Upavedas

The Upavedas are considered "applied knowledge" and refer to subjects of technicality. The four Upavedas are as follows:

Gandharvaveda: The study of aesthetics, including art, music, dance, poetry, and sculpture.

Dhanurveda: The science of archery and warfare.

Ayurveda: The science of health and life (the topic of this book!).

Sthapartaveda: The study of architecture and engineering.

Some schools consider Arthasastra the fourth Upaveda, instead of Sthapartaveda. Arthasastra is the science of policy, governance, and economics.

> **DEFINITION**
>
> The **Upavedas** are secondary Vedic teachings that go into four technical subjects—the arts, warfare, health, and architecture.

These studies are written about extensively, not only for their technical purposes but also as a means of transcendence. They are each considered important facets of civilization, from how to build structures to how to make art. The Vedas and Upavedas are extremely multidimensional texts that outline the importance of being well-rounded individuals and societies.

Shad Darshan: The Six Philosophies of Life

Ayurvedic philosophy is based on the Shad Darshan, the six Vedic philosophies of life. These philosophies are *Samkhya, Nyaya, Vaisheshika, Mimamsa, Yoga,* and *Vedanta.*

The first three philosophies, Samkhya, Nyaya, and Vaisheshika, are concerned with the physical world—how we heal the body and relate to the outside world. The latter three, Mimamsa, Yoga, and Vedanta, relate to understanding the inner realm and how we can evolve consciously. According to Ayurveda, true health lies in the balance between the two—physical and spiritual, inner and outer. All six philosophies lead to self-realization, just in different ways. It's important to know about Shad Darshan while studying Ayurveda because it illustrates that we should be just as concerned with the outside world as the inside world.

> **WISDOM OF THE AGES**
>
> The Shad Darshan philosophy contains the concept of *Purusha,* which means "city." Your body is believed to be a city with many houses, which are your body parts. You are not just comprised of individual, unrelated limbs and organs, but rather an entire city, with all these houses interconnected to make you a whole.

The Mind-Body Connection

The mind-body connection is a cornerstone of Ayurveda. Whatever happens in the body is reflected in the mind and vice versa. A patient cannot be treated based on a single symptom but rather the individual must be looked at as a whole. All the houses in the city are interrelated, and if one is out of electricity, the others will go in overdrive to make up for it. This is why it's important to be sure all parts of your being are functioning properly.

The Three Doshas and the Five Elements That Create Them

Ayurveda is based on the natural elements found on Earth, the elements we see, feel, and hear around us: fire, water, earth, air, and ether (space). We have all experienced each of these elements.

These elements exist not only in the planet, but also in your body, where they represent different components of your physical and mental characteristics. Fire is hot and powerful, while water is fluid and cool. Earth is dense and grounding, while air is light and moving. Ether is the one you can't see but can feel. It's the vastness of looking up at the stars on a clear day. It's your intuition.

Ayurveda uses these elements as references to explain all aspects of your physical and mental well-being. Each of us is born with a certain amount of these elements—some people are more fiery while others are more watery. If you've ever read your horoscope, they, too, relate to various elements, such as fire signs and earth signs.

However, Ayurveda takes a more scientific approach to the elements. It sees air as the movement of gas in your colon. It sees earth as your body compositing fat. It sees fire as your metabolism breaking down your food. It sees water as the hydration running through your cells. It sees ether as the space in your gastrointestinal tract. By understanding these elements, you can unlock hidden dimensions of your physical and emotional well-being.

These five elements make up the three Doshas—*Vata, Pitta,* and *Kapha.* These Doshas are energies used to describe your food, body, mind, environment, and everything else. Let me explain a bit more about what they are.

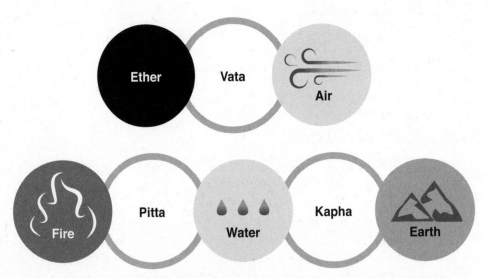

Vata is comprised of ether and air, while Pitta is comprised of fire and water, and Kapha is made up of water and Earth.

Vata: Air and Ether

The first Dosha is *Vata,* comprised of air and ether. It is dry, light, cold, rough, and mobile, just like air and ether energies. It is predominantly in your small intestines, colon, bones, pelvic area, belly button, heart, and head.

Vata is in charge of movement in the body, including the heartbeat, gastrointestinal tract, lungs, and diaphragm. Vata governs blood circulation; elimination of feces, urine, and sweat; respiration; ingestion; communication; heart function; menstruation; orgasm; hearing; touch; creativity; emotions; the nervous system; peristalsis and enzyme secretion; nutrient assimilation; and exercise and all other physical movement.

When Vata is out of balance, you experience symptoms in these areas. Examples in the body include poor blood circulation, feeling cold all the time, respiratory issues, heart palpitations, hearing problems, loss of senses, osteoporosis, and arthritis. Examples in the digestive system include constipation, bloating, gas, discomfort after eating, loss of appetite, low stomach acid, and inability to assimilate nutrients from foods. Examples in the pelvic area include amenorrhea (lack of menstruation), inability to orgasm, vaginal dryness, loss of interest in sex, and infertility. Examples in the mind include insomnia, anxiety, flakiness, indecisiveness, moodiness, dementia, Alzheimer's, loss of memory, forgetfulness, lack of creativity, nervous impulses, mental instability, fatigue, and restlessness.

> **DEFINITION**
>
> **Vata** is comprised of air and ether elements, regulating your nervous system and all movements within your body. When Vata is out of balance, you experience constipation, bloating, anxiety, irregular periods, and other related issues.

Pitta: Fire and Water

The second Dosha is *Pitta,* comprised of fire and water. It is hot, sharp, oily, liquid, and light, just like fire and water. It is predominantly in your stomach, small intestines, blood, liver, gallbladder, and spleen.

Pitta is in charge of transformation in the body, including digestion, metabolism, and nutrient absorption. Pitta works in your body as digestive enzymes in your small intestines and hydrochloric acid/pepsin in your stomach, helping your body break down food. Pitta is also present in your liver as bile and in your blood as hemoglobin. Your body releases excess Pitta through your sweat, which is why it's important to sweat regularly to release built-up Pitta. Pitta also governs metabolism, digestion, appetite, assimilation of nutrients, thirst, taste, vision, body temperature, luster of skin and hair, food and skin sensitivities, intelligence, courage, ambition, and determination.

When Pitta is out of balance, you experience symptoms in these areas. Examples in the body include feeling hot all the time, excess and/or foul-smelling sweat, early balding or graying hair, poor eyesight, excess bile, liver malfunctions, light sensitivity, and yellow eyes or skin. Examples in the digestive system include diarrhea, hyperacidity, heartburn, acid reflux, and ulcers.

Examples in the mind include anger, frustration, narcissism, competitiveness, stress, burnout, irritability, hatred, and impatience.

> **DEFINITION**
>
> **Pitta** is comprised of fire and water elements, governing your stomach and all transformations within your body. When Pitta is out of balance, you experience heartburn, overheating, anger, impatience, and other related issues.

Kapha: Earth and Water

The third Dosha is *Kapha,* comprised of earth and water. It is heavy, slow, cold, oily, soft, dense, and liquid, just like earth and water. It is predominantly in your lungs, stomach, pancreas, plasma, lymph system, joints, sinuses, nose, and tongue.

Kapha is in charge of structure in the body, including bone density, fat regulation, strength, and stamina. Kapha is like the earth, providing stability and support for your body, holding you together. Kapha has a lubricating quality, relieving friction between the cells and organs. It's present in your joints and muscles, making you strong. All bodily fluids, such as saliva and mucus, are related to Kapha. Kapha also governs lubrication, structure, energy, growth, stability, repair and restoration (including sleep), mucus, body mass and fat, moisture, grounding, nurturance, memory retention, kindness, and giving.

When Kapha is out of balance, you experience symptoms in these areas. Examples in the body include feeling cold all the time, clammy hands, weight gain, lethargy, mucus buildup, white-coated tongue, asthma, phlegm, infections, swelling, and water retention. Examples in the digestive system include slow metabolism, heaviness after meals, slow and sticky stools, and bloating. Examples in the mind include laziness, depression, loneliness, longing, sadness, jealousy, and attachment.

> **DEFINITION**
>
> **Kapha** is comprised of earth and water elements, governing your bone density and all structure within your body. When Kapha is out of balance, you experience heaviness, fatigue, water retention, depression, and other related issues.

We Are All the Doshas

The three Doshas are the building blocks for all matter—food, people, environments, and everything else. The more you become aware of the Doshas, the more you'll be able to see the interconnectivity of your own body. In Chapter 4, I help you determine which Dosha is most prevalent in you.

Keep in mind each of us has all three Doshas and all five elements within us. They all govern specific functions of your body, and without one, you would be left imbalanced. Some of us have a certain Dosha more predominant than another, which is why we may experience an imbalance in that Dosha. I want you first to be aware of how Dosha functions in your body before you try to figure out which one you are because really, you are all three. Without all the Doshas, your body would not function. They work with one another, in cooperation, and their imbalances affect one another.

Ayurveda is not a myth, theory, superstition, or religion but rather an intricate inner and outer scientific system that uses these elements to better understand the human body and psyche. The more comfortable you become with this terminology, the better you can understand the world you live in. Instead of looking at gas, you can look at excess air. Instead of looking at a rash, you can call it excess fire. Once you are aware of the elemental relations of each of your imbalances, you can connect them to other symptoms you may not have realized were interconnected. Each of these Doshas has a specific role in the larger machine, your human form.

The mind and body are interconnected, so a physical imbalance in a certain Dosha may lead to a mental disparity and vice versa. Pay close attention to how the mental and physical imbalances of the Dosha are interconnected and observe if any relate to you.

The Least You Need to Know

- Ayurveda is one of the four Upavedas, or technical Vedic sciences. The others include the arts, warfare, and architecture.
- Ayurveda is based on the five elements—air, ether, fire, water, and earth—which comprise the three Doshas—Vata, Pitta, and Kapha.
- Vata is comprised of air and ether. It controls the nervous system and all movement in the body.
- Pitta is comprised of fire and water. It operates the stomach and all transformation in the body.
- Kapha is comprised of earth and water. It regulates the structure and all stability in the body.
- You are a combination of all three Doshas but in varying amounts.

Your Unique Mind-Body Type

In Part 2, I walk you through a Dosha quiz to discover your Dosha and review the physical and mental characteristics of each Dosha in simple terminology that will finally make sense. I then take it a step further and show you how the Dosha you have today may be different from the one you were born with—and that's where your imbalances come from. I also offer some dietary, lifestyle, and even yoga and meditation advice specific to your Doshic constitution.

Discovering Your Dosha

For many people, this is their favorite part about Ayurveda—discovering your Dosha! As mentioned earlier, there are three Doshas—Vata, Pitta, and Kapha—and they are comprised of the five elements—air, ether (space), fire, water, and earth. Although you have all these elements within you, you were born with varying amounts.

The Doshas show up in all your characteristics, from the way you digest to the way you sleep. Each Dosha governs a specific function that affects the rest of your body. A Vata has a lot of airy characteristics in their body, such as bloating and restless thoughts. A Pitta has excess heat throughout their body, including increased body temperature and temper problems. A Kapha has substantial grounding in their body, from heaviness to laziness.

Why is it important to know your Dosha? Because your unique version of health is going to depend on your specific constitution. The following quiz helps you discover yours.

In This Chapter

- Discovering your Dosha
- Understanding your Dosha quiz results
- Dosha mental and physical traits
- The biggest obstacles for each Dosha

Dosha Quiz

I'm going to ask you some questions to help you determine your current Doshic balance. Remember, you are not entirely one Dosha but rather a combination of all three in varying amounts. This quiz helps you determine your primary, secondary, and tertiary Doshas.

Try to answer these questions honestly, rather than how you *wish* you were. If you have a difficult time answering these questions, ask a friend or loved one who knows you well to help you. They might be able to answer more objectively for you. The goal, however, is to know thyself.

1. Which most accurately describes your body?

   a. Naturally thin, lanky, slender

   b. Medium built, good muscular build

   c. Curvy, bigger built

2. How easily do you gain weight?

   a. Next to impossible; have to remember to eat to try not to lose any more weight

   b. Moderately; can lose or gain weight if I really try and can put on muscle easily

   c. Too easily; put on weight just by looking at food and have a hard time losing it

3. What are your eyes like?

   a. On the smaller side and actively moving

   b. Have a penetrating, deep gaze

   c. Big and beautiful

4. What is your skin like?

   a. Tends to get dry, quite thin, has visible veins

   b. Oily, acne-prone, has a reddish tint

   c. Moist, smooth, thick, combination

5. What is your hair like?

   a. Dry, frizzy, prone to split ends and breakage

   b. Fine, oily, tendency toward thinning or graying

   c. Thick, abundant, more on the oily side

6. What are your joints like?

   a. Prominent, tend to crack, often aching, injury-prone

   b. Flexible, agile

   c. Large, well padded

7. What is your digestion like?

   a. Variable—sometimes good, sometimes bad

   b. Strong and powerful

   c. Slow and weak

8. What is your elimination like?

   a. Tends toward constipation

   b. Regular, tends toward loose stools

   c. Thick, long, sluggish

9. Which digestive imbalances do you feel most?

   a. Bloating and gas

   b. Heartburn and acidic stomach

   c. Heaviness after eating and water retention

10. How is your body temperature?

    a. Always cold; prefer hot weather

    b. Usually warm; prefer cool weather

    c. Pretty adaptable; don't like cold, wet weather though

11. What is your temperament like?

    a. Enthusiastic, vivacious, creative

    b. Driven, passionate, ambitious

    c. Easy-going, giving, patient

12. What are your negative traits?

    a. Anxious, fearful, and/or nervous

    b. Competitive, aggressive, and/or impatient

    c. Lonely, depressed, and/or jealous

13. How do you sleep?

    a. Difficulty falling asleep, wake up often

    b. Moderate and sound

    c. Deep and long

14. How is your memory?

    a. Quick to remember, quick to forget

    b. Medium but accurate with facts

    c. Hard time remembering but then sustained

15. How are you with money and material possessions?

    a. Impulsive shopper; buy things and forget about them

    b. Calculated shopper; spend on luxuries that are worth it

    c. Hoarder; have a hard time letting things go

16. What subjects are you most drawn toward?

    a. The arts, spirituality, philosophy, literature, big-picture stuff

    b. Business, science, law, engineering, calculated stuff

    c. Counseling, teaching, human resources, care-giving, hands-on stuff

Dosha Quiz Results

Now count how many a, b, and c answers you got. A answers represent Vata, air, and ether. B answers represent Pitta, fire, and water. C answers represent Kapha, earth, and water.

The Dosha with the highest number is your *primary* Dosha. The Dosha with the second-highest number is your *secondary* Dosha. The Dosha with the lowest number is your *tertiary* Dosha. You may be about the same in two different categories, and that's totally fine. Most of us are dual-Doshas and our secondary Dosha changes throughout the course of our lives, according to our diet, age, season, exercise level, and other factors, which I discuss in Chapter 5.

I'm sure you're dying to know more about your results, so let's look at each of the Doshas in a little more detail.

AYURVEDIC ALERT

Keep in mind this self-assessment gives you a rough guideline on what your Doshic constitution is. It is not entirely accurate because there might be elements in your underlying physiology you're unaware of. The best way to truly determine your Doshic constitution is by consulting with an Ayurvedic practitioner.

Vata Characteristics

Physically, Vatas are the kinds of people who can eat whatever they want and never gain an ounce. In fact, they often are trying to gain weight but have a hard time putting on fat and muscle. Vatas are naturally small-boned, with prominent joints that often crack. They're often extremely tall or short, like a runway model or a ballerina. They have dry bodies, hair, skin, and nails. They often need braces to straighten their naturally crooked teeth, and if you look at their mouths, you'll notice their gums are on the thin side. They easily get dark circles under their eyes because their skin is so thin. They rarely sweat and often feel cold. They often experience back problems and have bone abnormalities, such as scoliosis or bunions.

Mentally, Vatas are extremely creative. They are interested in the arts, literature, spirituality, philosophy, and anything else that allows them to think outside the box. They talk quickly and have a million ideas in their heads. However, they can be very indecisive and change their minds frequently. They have a restless energy and tend to overanalyze things. They are prone to nervous system issues like anxiety, nervousness, and panic attacks.

If this sounds exactly like you, you are a Vata. You may be more Vata in your mind or in your body, so take note of that!

Pitta Characteristics

Physically, Pittas are the kind of people who gain muscle definition from a single workout. They are naturally athletic with medium-built bodies—not too big and not too lanky. They tend to have more oily hair that often goes gray or starts balding at an early age. Their skin is similarly oily, with a tendency toward breakouts. Both their hair and their skin often have a reddish tint. They sweat profusely and become overheated easily, which is why they need air-conditioning. They may have freckles, moles, and/or skin that burns easily in the sun. They are prone toward rashes, rosacea, and/or psoriasis.

Mentally, Pittas are very driven. They are interested in business, law, finance, fitness, science, and anything else that's achievement-oriented. They have organized minds and do well with structure. They are naturally domineering and tend to take positions of leadership, like the CEO of a Fortune 500 company. Sometimes that drive can become excessive. They can be controlling, demanding, and impatient with others. They are prone toward burnout and adrenal fatigue due to their perfectionist mentalities.

If this sounds like you, you are a Pitta.

If you have the characteristics of both a Pitta and a Vata, you are a Pitta-Vata or Vata-Pitta, depending on which you scored more in.

Kapha Characteristics

Physically, Kaphas are the kind of people who gain weight just by watching someone else eat. They are naturally bigger-boned with round faces and bodies. However, they have thick, moist hair; smooth, baby-soft skin; and long, lustrous nails. They maintain their body temperature well but prefer warm, dry weather. They tend to have cold, clammy hands and sugar cravings.

Mentally, Kaphas are very compassionate. They are interested in teaching, human resources, nursing, therapy, and anything else service-based. They are people-pleasers and often put the needs of others before their own. They are calm and peaceful, but have a tendency to be slow and resistant to change. They often hold on to the past and become depressed due to emotional eating and weight gain.

If this sounds just like you, you are a Kapha.

If you have a bit of the Vata type thrown in there, you are a Kapha-Vata or Vata-Kapha, depending on which you scored higher in.

If you are mixed with the Pitta type, you are a Kapha-Pitta or Pitta-Kapha, depending on your results.

If you are totally equal in all three, then congratulations, you are *tridoshic,* which is extremely rare. Or it could be that you think you are tridoshic, but really just have imbalances in all three Doshas, which is much more likely.

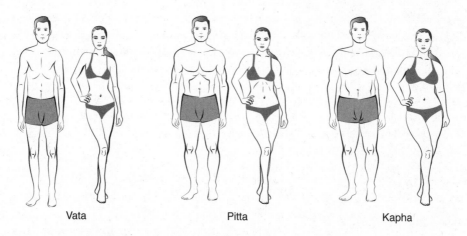

Vata   Pitta   Kapha

Vatas have slender bodies and a difficult time putting on muscle. Pittas have average-sized bodies and gain muscle easily. Kaphas have bigger-boned bodies and gain weight easily.

Making Sense of the Doshas

Now that you know about the Doshas and have somewhat figured out where you stand, let's relate them to other people. This way, you'll be able to spot Vatas, Pittas, and Kaphas in your family, in your circle of friends, and in public and better make sense of these Doshas.

Each Dosha is at risk for specific imbalances, which I make you aware of so you can continue to live a healthy and happy life by balancing your Doshas.

Lastly, it's totally possible to be facing an imbalance related to another Dosha. You will face imbalances related to all three Doshas at some point in your life, as we are all a combination of all three Doshas in varying amounts. In this section, I explain how you can have a predominant Dosha your entire life yet still sometimes relate to another specific Dosha from time to time.

Vata Types

Mentally, Vata types are quick and creative. They're always on the move and thinking of the next big thing. They get bored easily if they're in one place for too long. They can't sit still and are always looking for a challenge. They're big-picture people and see things others often do not. Examples of Vata types include Steve Jobs and Picasso. Any artist, writer, philosopher, or visionary would be an example of a Vata.

Physically, Vatas are the types of people who are always moving. You may notice they're often shaking their legs and can't sit still. They may pace to think and don't do well in a cubicle. They need a constant change of surroundings to stay stimulated. If you have a friend who just can't sit through a movie or is always getting up to walk around, he or she is a Vata.

The obstacle for Vatas is that all this movement in their minds can sometimes go haywire. They don't know how to put a stop to their thoughts. They go from brainstorming genius ideas to over-analyzing pointless situations, repeating conversations in their heads. This makes them easily distracted, and they sometimes can go off on tangents.

Just as easily as Vatas think of an idea, they lose it. They have a hard time remembering their own thoughts. In fact, their short-term memory often suffers because they are off in their own heads. Meditation can feel next to impossible for them. When they are sitting still, sometimes anxiety creeps in. They start to worry about things they don't need to think about. In general, their minds are in the future. The biggest task for them is to settle their minds and become present.

We all have our Vata moments—we're overwhelmed, anxious, and a little stuck in our heads. It's normal to feel this way at times because we live in a Vata-centric society. Most of us are multi-tasking and doing 12 things at once. This makes it especially difficult for us to stay centered.

When you feel this way, it's important for you to ground down and pacify your Vata, or lessen your Vata energy. You don't have to be a Vata type to feel anxious. It just means you currently have a Vata imbalance. I explain things you can do to fix this in Chapter 8.

However, some people just are more prone toward feeling this way, and those are the Vata types. They have an especially hard time staying grounded and are often very flighty, moody, and changeable. They're extremely sensitive to their environments and even a sound can disrupt them. These types must pay particular attention to pacifying their Vata because they are more at risk of feeling the side effects.

 WISDOM OF THE AGES

Here's a snapshot of Vata types:

Vata mind: Creative

Vata body: Lean

Vata obstacle: Sticking to one idea

Vata imbalance: Anxiety, digestive trouble

Pitta Types

Mentally, Pitta types are ambitious and hard-working. They're very focused and complete one task before starting another. They are strong leaders who do well in management. They have very organized minds and work on a schedule. They are able to follow through with tasks, no matter how much effort it takes. Examples of Pitta types include Warren Buffet and Kobe Bryant. Any manager, professional athlete, lawyer, or financial analyst would be an example of a Pitta.

Physically, Pittas are the types of people who need a good workout. They have a great deal of fire energy within them that needs to be released. They love to physically exhaust their bodies and use their muscles. They are naturally competitive and do well in sports, boot camps, marathons, and other athletic endeavors. If you have a friend who does triathlons for fun and has their entire month on a schedule, he or she is a Pitta.

The obstacle for Pittas is that all this fire in their bodies can transform into fire within their minds. They may become angry when things don't go their way and impatient when others take too long to perform a task. Pittas expect everyone else to put in as much effort as they do. They hold themselves at a very high standard and demand others to do the same. Pittas can be seen as intimidating for this reason.

Pittas also are prone to burnout because they don't know how to take a rest. All the fire within them begins to burn them from within. They are so used to having a great deal of energy that they oftentimes overpass their limits. They have difficulty seeing the benefits of taking it easy and want to get as much done as they can, and *now*. This causes their mental health to suffer, leaving them prone to adrenal fatigue. The biggest task for Pittas is to take things slow and cool down.

We all have Pitta energy within us—sometimes we're on a roll, going from one task to the next. In fact, it can feel addictive to achieve. However, if we keep going at that pace without any rest, we are at risk of exhaustion. This is when breakdowns happen.

The mind and body cannot always be operating at 100 miles per hour. It's important you take some time to relax and rejuvenate. Even if you are not a Pitta type, you have times in your life when you feel this way. You are in the groove, taking on more and more responsibilities until suddenly, they become too much. You notice you have less patience and are snapping at those around you more often. You may even crash, or blow up, like an erupting volcano. These are Pitta moments.

Then there are those who seem to be like this all the time. Their whole life is one giant to-do list, from one project to the next. They don't know how to schedule downtime into their busy schedules. To them, time is money, and it better not be wasted. And if you try to get them to stop, they'll bite.

It's extra important for Pitta types to settle down and take it easy because if they don't, they're at risk of losing their friends and loved ones—especially more sensitive Vata and calm Kapha types.

> **WISDOM OF THE AGES**
>
> Here's a snapshot of Pitta types:
>
> **Pitta mind:** Ambitious
>
> **Pitta body:** Athletic
>
> **Pitta obstacle:** Burnout
>
> **Pitta imbalance:** Anger, heartburn

Kapha Types

Mentally, Kapha types are peaceful, patient, and easy-going. They take their time but do a thorough job. They are natural caregivers and tend to the needs of those around them, often before their own. Their kindness is their strength, and they go out of their way to please their loved ones. They are extremely loyal and keep their friendships and relationships for the long haul. They thrive with people in one-on-one scenarios and make great listeners and counselors. They work well with their hands and enjoy tasks like cooking, gardening, or design. Patience is their virtue. Kaphas are extremely reliable and can always be counted on for support. If you have a friend who always puts others' needs before their own, he or she is a Kapha. Examples of Kapha types include Oprah Winfrey and Rachel Ray. Any caregiver, hospitality worker, therapist, schoolteacher, or nurse would be an example of a Kapha.

Physically, Kaphas are often complimented on their big eyes, full lips, and angelic voices, like Adele or Beyoncé. They naturally have curvy bodies, but at the same time, they have the strongest stamina of the Doshas. However, when they are out of balance, they allow their sedentary nature to take over and resist exercise, causing them to feel heavier and gain weight. This is why it is crucial for them to stay active to maintain balance.

The obstacle for Kaphas is that they're so busy ensuring everyone else is okay, they forget to take care of themselves. They listen to others' problems but have a hard time voicing their own. They may put a smile on their faces, but deep down, they harbor a sadness within. They feel like they have to be there to support others but have no one to take care of them. Sometimes, they feel totally alone, although they'll never let it show. Kaphas often overeat and become overweight due to this prolonged sadness.

Kaphas are prone toward depression because this longstanding sorrow begins to eat them alive. They isolate themselves from others and put this grief upon themselves because they do not want to burden others with their problems. Unlike Vatas, who have to tell everyone what's going on, and Pittas, who erupt at others but then get over it, Kaphas hold things within themselves. This makes them become heavier, with both weight and emotional grief.

We all may have undergone a time when we felt the Kapha blues. Nothing excited us anymore, and we wanted to stay in bed all the time and turn our backs on the rest of the world. It's normal to go through periods like this, and it happens to the best of us. However, it's important to bounce back by stimulating our bodies and minds to regain Pranic life force.

WISDOM OF THE AGES

Exercise is extremely medicinal to combat excess Kapha energy. Although it seems like a difficult task to exercise when you're feeling down, it's crucial to stimulate the body to stimulate the mind. A heavy body leads to heavy thoughts. To create lightness in the mind, you must create lightness in the body through movement and a light diet.

Then there are those who may have felt this way their entire lives. They don't know what it's like to wake up in the morning bustling with energy because they have always felt this heaviness. It's particularly important for Kaphas to stay active and mentally stimulated so they don't become dispirited and idle. They may have a hard time getting out of their comfort zones, but that's how they grow. To cultivate more creative Vata and ambitious Pitta in their lives, they need to start leading more active, dynamic lifestyles. The ideas will flow once the mind and body have been set in motion.

WISDOM OF THE AGES

Here's a snapshot of Kapha types:

Kapha mind: Peaceful

Kapha body: Rounded

Kapha obstacle: Putting others before self

Kapha imbalance: Depression, weight gain

The Least You Need to Know

- Although you have all three Doshas inside you, you have a primary, secondary, and tertiary Dosha. You may relate more to a specific Dosha in your mind and another in your body.
- Those with Vata bodies are naturally small-boned with dry skin and prominent joints. Those with Vata minds are quick and creative thinkers, prone to overthinking and anxiety.
- Those with Pitta bodies are medium built, well muscled, and have oily skin. Those with Pitta minds are passionate and sharp thinkers, prone to impatience and anger.
- Those with Kapha bodies are bigger built, curvy, and have moist skin. Those with Kapha minds are patient and compassionate thinkers, prone to depression and loneliness.
- The best way to know your unique constitution is by consulting with an Ayurvedic practitioner.

Qualities of the Doshas

Now that you've read Chapter 4 and have an understanding of the Doshas and which relate to you, let's dive further into each of their qualities.

Each Dosha has various attributes that associate with mental and physical traits. In this chapter, I break down these characteristics and then ask you a series of questions so you can see which relate to you. You may connect to qualities of more than one Dosha because they often overlap. For example, water is present in both Pitta and Kapha, so both have oily characteristics.

Keep in mind that you are not stuck with the qualities you were born with. The choices you make influence the way you are today, including your weight, skin, hair, digestion, and energy levels. After assessing what qualities you have, I give you more questions to help you determine how your dietary and lifestyle choices affect these characteristics. Are you ready to dive in?

In This Chapter

- A look at the qualities of each Dosha
- Assessing which attributes relate to you
- Balancing Doshic qualities with your diet and lifestyle
- Evaluating how your choices affect your body
- Addressing the underlying causes of your imbalances

Understanding the Doshas as Qualities

To really get a grasp of the Doshas, you must first understand them as elements. As mentioned in Chapter 4, the Doshas are made of the five elements—air, ether (space) fire, earth, and water. Here's how each are aligned:

Vata = air + ether

Pitta = fire + water

Kapha = earth + water

You were born with a certain amount of each element, but they change throughout your life due to the season, your diet, your stress level, your exercise habit, your emotional state, and a host of other factors.

Remember, Vatas have more airy, dry, and moving characteristics like dry skin, bloating, constipation, creative personalities, and desire to move. Pittas have more fiery, oily characteristics, including strong appetites and digestions, heartburn, loose stools, oily skin, strong personalities, and desire to achieve. Kaphas have more earthy, grounded characteristics such as a tendency toward weight gain, thick hair, sedentary bodies, and moist skin.

These are overall guidelines about what someone of only one Dosha is like. However, we are all a combination of the three Doshas, and our imbalances actually relate to specific qualities within each.

Each Dosha has a series of attributes, such as coldness, oiliness, or heaviness. Let's look at what each of these attributes are and what they mean for you. Then I ask you some questions so you can gauge your own.

Vata Attributes

Attribute	Manifestations in the Body
Dry	Dry skin, hair, lips, tongue; dry colon, tendency toward constipation; hoarse voice
Light	Light body frame, muscles, bones; scanty sleep
Cold	Cold hands, feet; poor circulation, hates cold and loves hot weather; body stiffness; menstrual irregularities
Rough	Rough bumps on skin, callused feet; cracked nails; rough hair; cracking joints
Subtle	Subtle twitching; delicate features; anxiety; muscle tremors

Attribute	Manifestations in the Body
Mobile	Mobile, flexible bodies; quick-moving, fast walker and talker; multitasker, constantly moving; moving eyes; many dreams, often about fleeing or flying; loves travel, can't stay in one place for too long; mood swings, uncertainty, changes mind easily
Clear	Intuitive, clear and open mind, philosophical, needs space to think
Astringent	Dryness in throat; burps, gets hiccups easily; loves moist and mushy food; craves sweet, sour, and salty food

Which relate to you?

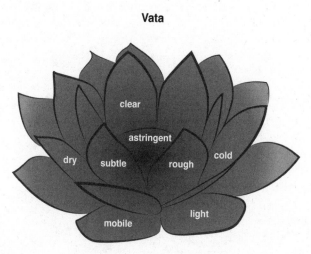

Vata

Pitta Attributes

Attribute	Manifestations in the Body
Hot	Strong digestive fire and appetite; high body temperature; doesn't do well in heat and humidity; goes gray/loses hair early; acne; inflammation
Sharp	Sharp mind, teeth, jaw line; penetrating gaze, pointed nose, tapering chin; sharp memory, can recall facts well
Light	Sensitive to bright light; fair skin, light-colored eyes; agile body
Oily	Oily skin, tendency toward acne; oily hair; oily stool; digestion and hair made worse by deep-fried or oily foods, including nuts
Liquid	Tendency toward loose stools; excess sweat, thirst, and urination

continues

Pitta Attributes   (continued)

Attribute	Manifestations in the Body
Spreading	Acne, rashes, and inflammation spread around the body; desire to spread their name around the world
Sour	Sour stomach acid, acidic pH; sensitive teeth and skin; excess salivation
Bitter	Bitter taste in mouth; nauseated, vomits easily; bitter personality, cynical
Pungent	Heartburn, burning sensation in stomach and mouth; irritability, anger
Putrid	Foul-smelling odor in underarms, mouth, and feet

Which relate to you?

Pitta

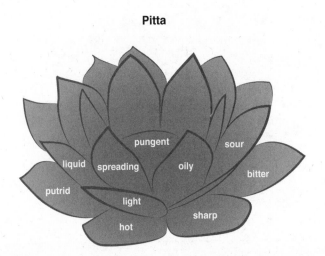

Kapha Attributes

Attribute	Manifestations in the Body
Heavy	Heavy feeling in body, bigger boned, tendency to become overweight, sedentary; heaviness in heart
Slow	Walks and talks slowly; slow digestion and metabolism; slow to initiate change
Cool	Cold body temperature; gets colds easily; cold digestive fire leading to slow metabolism; head colds
Oily	Tendency toward oily skin, hair, and stool; well-lubricated joints
Damp	Clammy hands; congestion in chest, sinuses, throat; headaches

Attribute	Manifestations in the Body
Smooth	Smooth skin and hair; smooth bowels; calm nature; smooth voice
Dense	Dense bodies, padding of fat around midsection, thick and dense legs; thick skin, hair, nails, and stool
Soft	Soft features, big eyes, soft skin and hair; compassionate, loving, gentle
Static	Sedentary, loves to sleep, sits many hours a day, habitual
Sticky	Loyal, loves to hug, attached; firm joints and organs; sticky stools
Cloudy	Often has cloudy mind, unable to think until after morning caffeine
Sweet	Craving for sweets; sweet personality; highly fertile, strong desire for sex and procreation
Salty	Retains water; long-standing energy; grows quickly; may crave salty foods

Which relate to you?

Kapha

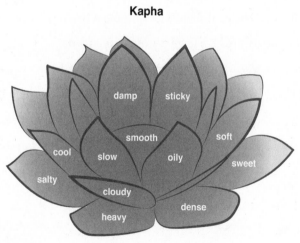

Your Qualities

Now that you have an understanding of the different qualities that make up the Doshas, where do you stand?

- Are you more cold or hot in nature?

- Are you more dry or oily?

- Are you more light or heavy?

- Are you more mobile or static?

- Are you more clear or sticky?

- Are you more rough or smooth?

These qualities, called the *gunas,* can help you better understand your body and the effects of the foods you put in it. There are 10 pairs of gunas, which I discuss more in Chapter 19.

In order to maintain health, you have to recognize your own subtle qualities and know what works for you. If you are naturally dry, putting dry foods in your body only heightens your imbalance, causing more dry skin and constipation. If you are naturally oily, eating fried or oily foods only worsens your acne and digestive issues. If you are naturally heavy, eating heavy foods only makes you want to hit the couch more.

Balancing Your Qualities

To balance these attributes, you must offset them with the opposite qualities:

- Vatas and Kaphas are both cold by nature, so they need warming foods.

- Pittas are hot by nature, so they need cooling, refreshing foods.

- Vatas are dry by nature, so they need more oily food.

- Pittas and Kaphas are oily by nature, so they need more drying and astringent foods.

- Vatas and Pittas are mobile by nature, so they need more grounding foods.

- Kaphas are dense by nature, so they need more light and stimulating foods.

- Vatas are rough by nature, so they need more creamy and soft foods.

- Kaphas are soft by nature, so they need more rough, fibrous foods.

- Pittas are sharp by nature, so they need more smooth foods.

- Vatas are more astringent by nature, so they need more sweet and salty foods.

- Pittas are more sour, bitter, and pungent by nature, so they need more sweet and astringent foods.

- Kaphas are more sweet and salty by nature, so they need more bitter, pungent and astringent foods.

In general, you must counterbalance your body's qualities with foods of the opposite quality so you reach equilibrium.

Your Choices Affect Your Characteristics

Knowing these basic qualities can help improve your health tremendously. They make it clear the impact of your external choices on your internal well-being.

Now, think about your own life and answer the following questions so you can assess how your choices are affecting the qualities of your body:

- Are the foods you eat more hot (like warm, cooked meals and soups) or cold (like salads, wraps, and snacks)?

- Are they more oily (like stir-fries and stews) or dry (like salads and crackers)?

- Are they more sweet (including all carbs), sour (like lemons), salty (like chips or seaweed), bitter (like brussels sprouts), pungent (like onions and garlic), or astringent (like chickpeas and cranberries)?

- Are the foods you eat more heavy (like steak, eggs, and potatoes) or light (like steamed vegetables and salads)?

- How does your body feel in general—more dense and heavy or mobile and light? How do you feel after meals?

- Is your lifestyle more active or sedentary?

- Is your skin more dry, oily, or smooth?

Addressing the Causes

These questions help you recognize how your dietary and lifestyle choices directly attribute to your bodily qualities. You might complain about acne but don't realize all the oils in your diet attribute to it. You might gain weight but don't think it's caused by your heavy diet. Now that you are aware, let's look at how you can counterbalance your excess qualities.

Dryness

If you noticed you have dry skin, hair, or nails and/or suffer from constipation and most of the foods you are eating are dry, that's your problem right there! You need more healthy oils in your diet to combat your dryness. Try cooking with sesame or coconut oil.

Dry foods: Crackers, chips, granola bars, cereal

Better choices: Stews, curries, stir-fries, avocados, nuts, healthy oils

Oiliness

If you have oily skin and hair and/or have heartburn and the majority of food you eat is oily, that's what you have to change. Decrease oils in your diet, including naturally oily nuts. Favor more leafy greens and cruciferous vegetables.

Oily foods: Oils, nuts, fried foods, tempura, stir-fries

Better choices: Steamed veggies, rice, fruits, oil-free curries and dressings

Heaviness

If you feel low in energy, have a hard time losing weight, and eat many heavy foods, that's your culprit. Try cutting fried foods and meat out of your diet and replace them with plant-based proteins like lentils and chickpeas. You don't gain more muscle the more protein you eat. Too much protein also contributes to fat. Kaphas require the least amount of protein in their diet because it makes them heavier and denser.

Heavy foods: Fried foods, meat, bread, pasta, eggs, stews

Better choices: Steamed veggies, salads, lentils, sprouts, seeds

 WISDOM OF THE AGES

Look at a food's qualities instead of calories. High-calorie foods are always heavy in quality. Instead of thinking, *This food is high in calories so I can't have it,* think *This food is heavy, and will make me feel heavy, so I don't want it.* Instead of placing restrictions on yourself, give yourself the option and choose not to have certain foods because of the way they make you feel.

Lightness

If you sometimes feel cold, dizzy, or forgetful and eat mostly cold, light foods like snacks or salads, that's your issue. Try adding more grounding foods into your diet, like root vegetables and stews, to offset your lightness. This is particularly important for Vatas, who have a tough time grounding.

Light foods: Popcorn, salads, smoothies, raw foods

Better choices: Sweet potatoes, squash, ginger, parsnips, soups, stews

Your diet and lifestyle play a huge role in the qualities within your body. You can offset your natural imbalances by making up for them in your diet and everyday life.

The first step is to understand the qualities within your body. Then, you can focus on the qualities of the foods you regularly consume. Finally, you can counterbalance your qualities with those in your food to create lasting health.

The Least You Need to Know

- Each Dosha has particular attributes that influence the body.
- Vata has cold, light, dry, rough, subtly mobile, and clear qualities.
- Pitta has hot, sharp, light, oily, smooth, damp, and sticky qualities.
- Kapha has heavy, slow, cool, oily, and damp qualities.
- To regain equilibrium, you must counterbalance these uneven qualities with your diet and lifestyle.

CHAPTER 6

The Best Foods for Each Dosha

By now you're probably wondering, *So what do I eat?* This is one of the most pressing issues in Ayurveda, and don't worry—Ayurveda has a lot of answers for you.

The foods you should eat are related to the Dosha in which you're imbalanced. Ayurveda has three separate guidelines for pacifying Vata, Pitta, and Kapha. In this chapter, I explain the best foods to eat, and what to avoid, to balance each Dosha.

You want to eat foods that stimulate your digestive fire, or agni. Within your body exists an internal flame in charge of breaking down your food and assimilating the nutrients. This is also referred to as your digestion or metabolism. To make the most of your meals, you should choose ingredients with nutrients you can easily assimilate. That's why Ayurveda recommends cooked vegetables in most situations. Cooked foods are easier for your body to break down compared with raw foods, making them a good option for those with weak digestive fires. You'll see me refer to the digestive fire throughout the book, so just know that it relates to your digestion and metabolism.

In This Chapter

- The best fruits, veggies, grains, dairy products, oils, and more for each Dosha
- Foods each Dosha should avoid
- Sample recipes for each Dosha

If you're confused about what to eat, choose foods good for the Dosha where your imbalance lies. For example, if you're cold and bloated, go for the Vata guidelines. If you're hot and acidic, go for the Pitta guidelines. If you're overweight and heavy, go for the Kapha guidelines.

The Best Foods for Vatas

Vatas are naturally cold, dry, mobile, and rough in energy so they need foods of the opposite qualities. That means more warm, moist, dense, and oily foods. These foods counterbalance their Vata characteristics, such as dry skin, bloating, gas, indigestion, anxiety, and insomnia, among others. Through diet, Vatas can completely change their negative qualities and regain balance.

Fruits

Vatas should favor fruits that are sweet and nourishing. They don't do as well with fruits that are overly bitter or astringent, like cranberries. They also should avoid dry fruit completely.

If a Vata's digestive system is compromised, fruit will make them very bloated and uncomfortable. In that case, they should have only cooked fruit, such as stewed apples, until their digestion is healed.

Consume fruits by themselves and 30 minutes before meals for optimal digestion.

Fruits Vatas can enjoy:

- Apples (cooked)
- Apricots (fresh)
- Avocados
- Bananas (ripe)
- Berries
- Cantaloupes/melons
- Cherries
- Coconuts
- Dates (fresh, cooked, or soaked)
- Figs (fresh, cooked, or soaked)
- Grapefruit
- Grapes
- Kiwifruits
- Lemons
- Limes
- Mangoes
- Oranges
- Papayas
- Peaches
- Pineapples
- Plums
- Watermelon (in hot weather only)

Fruits Vatas should avoid:

- Apples (raw)
- Bananas (green)
- Dates (dry)
- Dried fruit

Vegetables

Vatas do best with cooked vegetables because they are easier to digest. Raw vegetables have dry, rough, and cold qualities, which imbalance already dry, rough, and cold Vatas. Vatas should avoid raw vegetables until their digestive fire strengthens. Instead, they should favor root vegetables, which have grounding qualities.

If you are a Vata and choose to have a vegetable on the "vegetables Vatas should reduce" list, be sure it's well cooked with mustard seeds and sesame oil, which make it much easier to digest. If you do eat raw vegetables, do so in the middle of the day when your digestive fire is strongest.

> **AYURVEDIC ALERT**
>
> Love salads but a Vata type? Unfortunately, they're not the best thing for your digestion. Vata is a light, dry and airy energy, therefore needs more heavy, oily and Earthy foods to help balance it out. Leafy greens have the same qualities as Vata, therefore throw it off balance.

Vegetables Vatas should favor:

- Asparagus
- Beets
- Carrots (cooked)
- Chiles (small amounts)
- Cilantro
- Cucumbers
- Garlic
- Green beans
- Leeks
- Mustard greens
- Okra
- Olives (black)
- Onions (cooked)
- Parsnips
- Peas (cooked)
- Pumpkin
- Rutabagas
- Spinach (cooked)
- Squash (all types)
- Sweet potatoes
- Watercress
- Zucchini

Vegetables Vatas should reduce:

- Any raw vegetable, especially cruciferous

Grains

Vatas do very well with grains generally because they are easy to digest, grounding, and sweet in taste. They provide energy for the body and help balance hormones as well.

However, certain grains are better than others. Some grains, such as barley, have more cooling properties and aren't as nourishing for Vatas. Eating grains cooked and warm is much better for Vatas than eating them cold in a salad.

Grains Vatas should focus on:

- Amaranth
- Basmati rice
- Brown rice
- Oats (cooked, especially steel cut)
- Quinoa (any color)
- Sprouted wheat bread
- Wild rice

> **WISDOM OF THE AGES**
>
> Always soak your grains for optimal digestion. I just leave them in a bowl of water the night before I cook them and rinse them out before boiling. This little step results in easier to digest, more nutritious grains, as well as a shorter cooking time.

Grains Vatas should avoid:

- Any cold, dry, or puffed grain

Legumes

Legumes are great sources of protein, and they're much easier to digest than meat. However, some Vatas have very weak digestions and cannot tolerate many legumes without feeling bloated or gassy. Legumes also are astringent in taste, which can dry out Vatas.

Be sure legumes are well cooked and contain spices, particularly cumin, so they're easy to assimilate. Listen to your body, and notice how it reacts.

Easiest-to-digest legumes for Vatas:

- Mung daal (split mung beans)
- Tofu (served hot)

Beans that may make Vatas gassy:

- Any other type of bean

Dairy

Dairy products are recommended in Ayurveda, but dairy back then was very different from what it is now. 5,000 years ago, it was always raw and organic, coming straight from the neighborhood cow. Today, thanks to factory farming, our dairy products are no longer pure and contain hormones and other additives. On top of that, they are pasteurized, which kills their live enzymes and lowers many key nutrients, including vitamins C and E.

Thankfully, many dairy alternatives are available, such as flax, hemp, coconut, almond, rice and pea, which I recommend because they are completely plant based and hormone free. If you want to consume dairy products, be sure they're organic and free of recombinant bovine growth hormone (rGBH), a genetically engineered artificial hormone injected into dairy cows to make them produce more milk.

If possible, seek raw dairy products, which contain the enzymes and vitamins that make dairy products nutritious. Raw dairy products are easier to digest than their pasteurized counterparts and contain more vitamins, enzymes, and healthy bacteria. In fact, a quart of raw milk from grass-fed cows contains 50 percent more vitamin E than the same amount of pasteurized milk. Many vitamins, including vitamin C, are destroyed by heat, which is why pasteurized milks are fortified with synthetic vitamins. Your body does not absorb these laboratory-made vitamins in the same way as it does plant-based vitamins.

For optimal digestion, consume dairy at least 1 hour before any other food and do not combine it with fruit or meat.

Dairy Vatas should favor:

- Ghee (clarified butter)
- Goat's milk, cheese, or yogurt
- Kefir
- Yogurt (unsweetened)

Dairy Vatas should avoid:

- Frozen yogurt
- Ice cream
- Nonorganic products
- Powdered milk

Nuts and Seeds

Nuts and seeds make great snacks for Vatas. They are oily, heavy, and dense, counterbalancing Vatas' dry, light, and mobile energy. However, enjoy nuts in moderation because they can be too heavy for your digestive fire when eaten in excess.

Always choose raw and unsalted nuts. Almonds are considered the best nut for Vatas. For optimal digestion, soak almonds overnight in water and remove the skin before eating.

Nuts and seeds Vatas should incorporate:

- Any raw nut and seed

Nuts and seeds Vatas should avoid:

- Roasted, salted nuts

Animal Products

Vatas do the best with animal proteins compared to the other Doshas because they often need the strength. However, it is not necessary to incorporate animal products in your diet to rebalance Vata. Ayurveda recommends a mostly vegetarian diet, with the exception of those who are extremely weak or vigorously active. These are only guidelines if you choose to incorporate animal products in your diet.

Vatas should favor meats that are moist, sweet, and easy to digest. Stay away from those that are overly heavy or dry. Eggs and chicken should always be organic, fish should be wild caught, and meat should be grass fed to ensure you obtain the greatest amount of nutrients.

Animal products Vatas should favor:

- Beef
- Chicken or turkey (especially dark meat)
- Eggs (pasture-raised)
- Fish (fresh and saltwater)

Animal products Vatas should avoid:

- Lamb
- Pork
- Rabbit
- Turkey (white meat)
- Venison

Oils

Oils are very pacifying for Vatas because they offset their dry, rough bodies and colons. Vatas require the most amount of lubrication in their diets to promote regularity and hydration. Vatas should favor warming oils and avoid those that are too light, dry, or processed.

> **WISDOM OF THE AGES**
>
> Toxins concentrate in fats, so it's especially important to ensure your oil is organic and pure. Go for raw, unprocessed oils that aren't mixed with other, cheaper oils.

Oils Vatas should favor:

- Almond oil
- Extra-virgin pure olive oil
- Extra-virgin raw coconut oil
- Mustard oil
- Sesame oil

Oils Vatas should avoid:

- Canola oil
- Corn oil
- Palm oil
- Peanut oil

Sweeteners

Vatas do best with sweeteners because people of this Dosha are often underweight and need the extra calories. However, that doesn't mean all Vatas need to gain weight. If you're trying to manage your weight, it's best to avoid sweeteners and opt for plant-based sources of sugar, such as fruit.

Today, many natural alternative sweeteners are available, such as monk fruit sweetener, stevia, and birchwood xylitol. When Ayurveda was created 5,000 years ago, these choices did not exist and, understandably, were not written about in the traditional texts. However, you can still benefit from these sugar alternatives, which won't affect your blood sugar levels nor feed bad bacteria in your gut.

Most people unknowingly consume too much sugar in their diets, resulting in diabetes and other illnesses, so I recommend opting for nonglycemic sugar alternatives like monk fruit sweetener, stevia, and birchwood xylitol.

I added an asterisk (*) to the new sweetener alternatives that did not exist in Ayurvedic times so you can differentiate.

Sweeteners Vatas should favor:

- Birchwood xylitol*
- Coconut sugar
- Dates/date sugar
- Honey (raw, heated, cooked, or pasteurized)

- Maple syrup (in moderation)
- Monk fruit sweetener*
- Stevia (liquid, organic)*

Sweeteners Vatas should avoid:

- Cane juice or syrup
- White sugar

Spices

In Ayurveda, spices are viewed as medicine. They are especially great to stimulate Vatas' weak digestive fires.

However, *spices* don't necessarily mean *spicy*. In fact, overly spicy food is actually difficult for Vatas to digest because it's overstimulating and causes loose stools. It's best to spice your food with warming spices like ginger, cumin, and mustard seeds without making it overly hot. Vatas also should reduce spices that are overly drying or harsh, like those listed in the following "in moderation" list, unless for medicinal purposes.

Be sure your spices are pure, organic, and high quality. Many store-bought spices contain anticaking agents and fillers that can be harmful for your health.

Spices Vatas should favor:

- Ajwan
- Anise
- Asafoetida
- Basil
- Bay leaf
- Black pepper
- Cardamom
- Cinnamon
- Cloves
- Coriander (seeds or powder)
- Cumin (seeds or powder)
- Fennel
- Ginger (fresh or powder)
- Mustard seeds
- Nutmeg
- Paprika
- Rosemary
- Saffron
- Turmeric

Spices Vatas should use in moderation:

- Cayenne
- Chili powder
- Fenugreek
- Horseradish
- Neem

Sample Vata Recipe

Vatas need warming, grounding recipes to nourish their bodies and keep their digestive fires going. They do well with cooked hearty dishes such as curries and stews, rather than cold salads and light snacks, which throw them off balance. They also need the most protein of all the Doshas because they have a hard time retaining muscle and bone mass, which is why tofu is a great option for them.

Curried Coconut Tofu Curry Over Wild Rice

This is one of my favorite simple recipes for cool, dry Vata types. It is packed with flavor and fragranced with Ayurvedic spices warming a Vata's digestive fire from within. It also boasts protein-filled chunks of tofu satiating a Vata's flighty appetite, served over easily-digested wild rice. Best of all, you can put this dish together in under 30 minutes flat. It's so easy even an airy Vata can manage to complete it without losing interest.

1 TB. coconut oil	$1/2$ cup diced carrots
1 small yellow onion, diced	$1/2$ cup okra, lightly chopped
4 garlic cloves, minced (2 TB.)	2 TB. curry powder
1 TB. fresh grated ginger (or 1 tsp. ground)	2 cans full-fat coconut milk
	1 cup vegetable stock
$1/2$ 12.3 oz. pkg. extra-firm organic tofu, drained, pressed and cubed	$1/2$ tsp. sea salt
	$1/4$ tsp. black pepper

1. In a large saucepan or pot, heat 1 TB. coconut oil to medium heat. Add the chopped onion, minced garlic, ginger, diced tofu, carrot, okra, salt, and pepper. Allow to cook for 5 minutes, stirring frequently.

2. Add the curry powder, coconut milk, and veggie stock and stir-fry. Bring to a low simmer then reduce heat and continue cooking for 10-15 minutes as the curry thickens.

3. Remove from pot and serve over wild rice.

WISDOM OF THE AGES

Curry can commonly be bought at supermarkets but is actually a combination of the Ayurvedic spices cumin, coriander, turmeric, mustard seed, ginger and chili powder. Curry powder does not exist in India, as people typically make their own with the above spices.

The Best Foods for Pittas

Pittas are naturally hot, oily, sharp, and pungent in energy so they need foods that contain the opposite qualities. That means more cool, juicy, sweet, and dry foods. These cleansing ingredients counterbalance their natural Pitta characteristics, such as oily skin, heartburn, hyperacidity, impatience, overheating, and ulcers, among others. With an appropriate diet, Pittas can cool their minds and bodies to regain balance and inner peace.

Fruits

Pittas should favor fruits that are juicy, sweet, and astringent. They should avoid sour, acidic fruits like sour grapes and grapefruit. Some Ayurvedic sources say Pittas should avoid bananas because they can be too heating, but it depends on your personal digestion. Pittas tend to do well with most fruits due to their strong digestion. Keep in mind, the best fruit depends on the season. Go for organic whenever possible, especially those fruit whose skin you also eat, like apples and berries.

For optional digestion, consume fruits by themselves and 30 minutes before meals.

Fruits Pittas can enjoy:

- Apples (sweet)
- Apricots (sweet)
- Avocados
- Bananas (sweet)
- Berries (sweet)
- Cherries (sweet)
- Coconuts
- Dates/figs
- Grapes (red, purple, black)
- Mangoes (ripe)
- Melons
- Oranges (sweet)
- Papayas
- Pears
- Pineapples (sweet)
- Plums (sweet)
- Pomegranates
- Strawberries

Fruits Pittas should avoid:

- Excess sour fruits like grapefruit and lemon

Vegetables

Pittas should focus on sweet, bitter, and/or astringent vegetables. Although Ayurveda recommends eating mostly cooked vegetables, Pittas do best with raw vegetables because their digestive systems are so strong. If you do choose to consume raw foods, such as salads, it's best to have them for lunch when your digestive fire is at its peak and your body has the rest of the day to break down the fibrous cell walls.

Pittas need to avoid vegetables that are particularly pungent, heating, spicy, or sharp, such as garlic, chiles, and onions. They also should steer clear of nightshades, including tomatoes, eggplants, and peppers.

> **WISDOM OF THE AGES**
>
> Nightshade vegetables are especially harmful for Pittas' digestion. *Nightshades* is a term commonly used for the group of plants in the *Solanaceae* family. These plants contain glycoalkaloids, natural pesticides that fight against bacteria, fungi, viruses, and insects. Nightshade vegetables include tomatoes, eggplants, peppers, potatoes, paprika, goji berries, and tobacco. Even if you aren't a Pitta, if you're experiencing digestive issues, try removing these vegetables from your diet and see if your digestion improves.

Various Ayurvedic sources offer slightly different suggestions for what to include and avoid, so go with what works for your body.

Vegetables Pittas should favor:

- Artichokes
- Asparagus
- Beets (cooked)
- Bell peppers
- Broccoli
- Brussels sprouts
- Cabbage
- Carrots (cooked)
- Cauliflower
- Celery
- Cucumbers
- Leafy greens
- Spinach (raw)
- Sprouts (not spicy)
- Squash (all types)
- Sweet potatoes
- Zucchini

Vegetables Pittas should reduce or avoid:

- Daikon radishes
- Eggplants
- Garlic
- Green chiles
- Leeks (raw)
- Mustard greens
- Onions (raw)
- Peppers (hot)
- Radishes (raw)
- Tomatoes
- Turnips

Grains

Grains should be a staple in the Pitta diet and consumed in their most natural form. Pittas do well with grains because they provide fuel for their active bodies and have a sweet, nourishing taste that's easy to digest. Pittas should favor grains that are cooling, drying, and grounding in nature. Avoid heating grains and yeasted breads (that is, breads that rise).

Grains Pittas should go for:

- Amaranth
- Barley
- Couscous
- Oats
- Quinoa
- Rice (basmati, white, wild)
- Spelt
- Wheat

Grains Pittas should avoid:

- Buckwheat
- Corn
- Millet
- Polenta
- Rye
- Yeasted breads

Legumes

Legumes are wonderful for Pittas because they satisfy their need for protein in a plant-based way and are naturally astringent, cooling warm Pitta bodies. Stay away from canned, salted, heating, or fried legumes, which can cause toxic accumulation.

Legumes Pittas should choose:

- Black beans
- Chickpeas
- Lentils
- Mung daal (mung split beans)

- Split peas
- Tempeh
- Tofu

Legumes Pittas should minimize:

- Any canned beans
- Soy meat alternatives

- Soy sauce

Dairy

Dairy products were recommended in Ayurveda, but nowadays, we have many alternatives, such as almond or coconut milk, which are actually preferable for Pittas, who are particularly sensitive to toxins in dairy products, such as rGBH, mentioned earlier.

If you choose to consume dairy, opt for raw dairy products, which contain the enzymes that make dairy easier to digest. Be sure all dairy products are organic and free of hormones and other chemicals. For optimal digestion, consume dairy at least 1 hour before any other food and do not combine with fruit or meat.

Pittas should favor soft cheeses, rather than hard or aged cheeses, and avoid sour dairy products like sour cream and buttermilk

Dairy Pittas should favor:

- Butter (unsalted)
- Ghee

- Goat's milk, cheese, and yogurt
- Organic yogurt (unsweetened, homemade)

Dairy products Pittas should avoid:

- Butter (salted)
- Buttermilk
- Cheese (hard)

- Frozen yogurt
- Sour cream
- Yogurt (store-bought or with fruit)

Nuts and Seeds

Nuts are especially oily and cause an imbalance in Pittas, leading to acne. Seeds, however, are lighter and more favorable. Pittas should choose nuts and seeds that are more cooling in nature and always opt for raw and unsalted versions. For optimal digestion, soak almonds overnight in water and remove the skin before eating.

Nuts and seeds Pittas should incorporate:

- Almonds (soaked and peeled)
- Chia seeds
- Flaxseeds
- Pumpkin seeds
- Sunflower seeds

Nuts and seeds Pittas should reduce or avoid:

- Any nut besides soaked almonds

Animal Products

Pittas do best on a vegetarian diet because they are more sensitive to toxins and already hot in nature. Animal products are extremely heating and often contain hormones, antibiotics, and other toxins, which disrupt Pittas.

Keep in mind, too, that animal products aggravate Pittas and ideally should be kept to a minimum.

> **WISDOM OF THE AGES**
>
> It's your choice if you want to include animal products in your diet, and Ayurveda offers suggestions to follow if you make that decision. Pittas should favor light and dry meats and stay away from oily and heating products.

Animal products Pittas should favor:

- Chicken or turkey (white meat)
- Eggs (whites only)
- Fish (freshwater or salmon)

Animal products Pittas should avoid:

- Beef
- Chicken or turkey (dark meat)
- Eggs (yolks)
- Lamb
- Pork
- Shellfish

Oils

Pittas are oilier in nature and should not use excess oil in their diet. However, moderate amounts of oils are advisable because they do lubricate the body. Pittas should opt for oils that are lighter in quality and avoid processed oils, which are higher in toxins.

Oils Pittas should favor:

- Extra-virgin raw coconut oil
- Extra-virgin raw olive oil
- Flaxseed oil
- Ghee

Oils Pittas should avoid:

- Canola oil
- Corn oil
- Peanut oil
- Soy oil
- Sunflower oil

Sweeteners

Sweeteners are fine in moderation because the sweet taste helps balance Pittas. Excess, however, is heating and aggravating to Pittas. Go for sweeteners that have no impact on your blood sugar levels, such as monk fruit sweetener, stevia, and birchwood xylitol, which are less heating for the system.

Most people already have too much sugar in their diets so I recommend going for the nonglycemic sugars like monk fruit sweetener, stevia, and birchwood xylitol.

I added an asterisk (*) to the new sweetener alternatives that did not exist in Ayurvedic times so you can differentiate.

Sweeteners Pittas should favor:

- Birchwood xylitol*
- Coconut sugar
- Dates/date sugar
- Honey (raw)
- Maple syrup
- Monk fruit sweetener*
- Stevia (liquid, organic)*

Sweeteners Pittas should avoid:

- Brown sugar
- Cane sugar/syrup
- Honey
- Jaggary (noncentrifugal cane sugar)
- Molasses
- White sugar

Spices

Pittas love spicy foods because they stimulate their internal fire. However, it does throw them off balance. That said, Pittas can incorporate many spices in their meals, as long as they aren't overly spicy.

Pittas still can consume some heating spices, such as cumin, turmeric, and saffron, as long as they aren't super hot like chili powder and cayenne. Think *spices,* not *spicy.*

The best for Pittas, however, are cooling herbs.

Spices Pittas should favor:

- Basil (fresh)
- Black pepper (small amounts)
- Cardamom
- Cinnamon
- Coriander
- Cumin
- Dill
- Fennel
- Ginger (fresh)
- Mint
- Parsley
- Peppermint
- Saffron
- Turmeric
- Vanilla

Spices Pittas should reduce:

- Cloves
- Garlic
- Peppers

Sample Pitta Recipe

While Pittas may like their dishes hot and spicy, what they really need is something cooling and simple. Pittas do well with cruciferous vegetables, like broccoli or cauliflower, as well as airy leafy greens. They do best with simple meals to give their overactive digestive fires a chance to relax and refresh.

Cooling Chickpeas and Veggies Over Toasted Quinoa

1 TB. coconut oil

$1/2$ yellow onion, chopped

3 tsp. ground cumin

2 tsp. turmeric

$1/2$ tsp. ground cardamom

4 cups chopped cauliflower, broccoli, asparagus, squash, or zucchini (your choice)

2 cups chickpeas, cooked

$2^1/2$ cups water

2 tsp. sea salt

1 cup quinoa, (preferably soaked beforehand)

Optional fresh herbs as garnish

1. In a large pot over medium-high heat, heat 1 TB. coconut oil. Add the yellow onion with 1 teaspoon cumin, 1 teaspoon turmeric, and cardamom, and sauté for about 4 minutes or until golden brown.

2. Add veggies, chickpeas, ½ cup water, 1 teaspoon cumin, remaining 1 teaspoon turmeric, and sea salt. Cover, reduce heat to medium, and cook for 10 minutes, stirring occasionally.

3. Meanwhile, heat a large saucepan over medium heat, add quinoa, and toast for 1 to 2 minutes or until dry.

4. Add remaining 2 cups water, 1 teaspoon sea salt, and remaining 1 teaspoon cumin. Reduce heat to medium-low, cover, and cook for 15 to 20 minutes or until all liquid is absorbed. Remove from heat, allow cool for several minutes, and fluff with a fork.

5. Place quinoa on a plate, top with vegetable/chickpea mixture, and enjoy warm. Add fresh herbs on the side if you like.

WISDOM OF THE AGES

Cooling food doesn't necessarily mean a salad or smoothie. It is possible to prepare warm, cooked food with cooling qualities by using ingredients such as fresh herbs; chickpeas; coconut oil; and light, fluffy quinoa.

The Best Foods for Kaphas

Kaphas are naturally dense, heavy, oily, and sweet in energy so they need foods that contain the opposite qualities. That means more light, stimulating, dry, bitter, astringent, and pungent items. These foods restore their imbalances, such as lethargy, weight gain, swelling, mucus buildup, and sluggish metabolism. Through a well-balanced diet, Kaphas can gain energy and lose weight to regain balance.

Fruits

Kaphas should only have fruits that are light and minimally sweet or sour. Kaphas tend to gain weight easily, and the excess sugar in fruits can add up. Similarly, tropical fruits like bananas and mangoes are particularly sweet, heavy, dense, and watery, which add to Kaphas' imbalances. Kaphas should choose astringent fruit and only have one serving a day.

Go for organic whenever possible, especially on fruit whose skin you eat, like apples and berries.

For optimal digestion, consume fruits by themselves and 30 minutes before meals.

Fruits Kaphas should enjoy:

- Apples
- Apricots (fresh)
- Berries (all)
- Cherries
- Cranberries

- Lemons
- Limes
- Pears
- Pomegranates

Fruits Kaphas should avoid or minimize:

- Avocados
- Bananas
- Coconuts (meat)

- Dates
- Mangoes

Vegetables

Vegetables should be the center of Kaphas' diets because they are very cleansing. Those that are bitter, pungent, or astringent are the best for helping Kaphas reduce weight and uplift their bodies. Avoid vegetables that are heavy, dense, oily, or watery, such as heavy stews, mashed potatoes, tempuras, and oily stir-fries.

Kaphas have weak digestive systems, so it's best for them to lightly cook their vegetables, such as via steaming or roasting, to make them easier to digest. Avoid using excess oil, and try water-sautéing vegetables. It's best for Kaphas to avoid raw foods, but if you choose to consume them, they're best at lunch when your digestive fire is strongest and you have the rest of the day to break down the meal.

Vegetables Kaphas should favor:

- Artichokes
- Asparagus
- Beets
- Bell peppers
- Broccoli
- Brussels sprouts
- Cabbage
- Carrots
- Cauliflower
- Celery
- Leafy greens
- Peas
- Peppers (sweet and hot)
- Radishes
- Spinach
- Sprouts
- Turnips

Vegetables Kaphas should reduce:

- Olives
- Potatoes
- Pumpkins
- Squash

Grains

Kaphas should be mindful of their portions of grains because they're sweet and building and can cause weight gain. Grains should be light and dry in energy. Stay completely away from breads, pastas, and pastries.

Grains Kaphas should go for:

- Amaranth
- Barley
- Buckwheat
- Millet
- Quinoa

Grains Kaphas should avoid:

- Pasta
- Wheat

- White or brown rice
- Yeasted breads

Legumes

Legumes are great for Kaphas because they are astringent in taste, counterbalancing their natural sweetness. Kaphas should be sure their beans are well spiced, especially with cumin, to make them easier to digest.

Legumes Kaphas should choose:

- Black beans
- Chickpeas
- Lentils
- Mung daal (mung beans)

- Split peas
- Tempeh
- Tofu (served hot)

Legumes Kaphas should avoid:

- Kidney beans
- Miso
- Soy beans

- Soy cheese
- Soy sauce
- Tofu (served cold)

Dairy

Kaphas are naturally attracted to cheese and ice cream, but it's the worst thing for them. Kapha types should avoid dairy products because they're heavy and cooling, just like Kapha energy. Like increases like, and Kaphas need to stay away from anything that makes them more heavy, dense, and cold.

Some Kaphas can digest goat milk products without a problem because they contain less lactose and are lighter in energy. However, nondairy milk is still the best option. I recommend unsweetened coconut, almond, or pea milk.

Nuts and Seeds

Nuts are heavy, dense, and oily and cause an imbalance in Kaphas. The only nuts Kaphas can have are soaked and peeled almonds, and even those should be consumed in moderation. Seeds are always a better, lighter option for Kapha types.

Nuts and seeds Kaphas should choose:

- Almonds (soaked and peeled)
- Chia seeds
- Flaxseeds
- Hemp seeds
- Pumpkin seeds
- Sunflower seeds

Nuts and seeds Kaphas should reduce or avoid:

- Excess nuts and nut butters

Animal Products

Kaphas should not incorporate too many animal products in their diet because these foods are particularly heavy in property, increasing Kapha. Excess protein can cause Kaphas to gain fat because they don't require as much protein as the other Doshas. It is totally possible for Kaphas to get all the protein they need from a plant-based diet, and this is recommended actually.

However, if you choose to consume animal products as a Kapha, select those that are light and dry. Eat animal products only in small amounts and infrequently. Be sure all products are organic and preferably from a local farmer.

Animal products Kaphas should favor:

- Chicken or turkey (white meat)
- Eggs (pasture-raised)
- Fish (freshwater)

Animal products Kaphas should avoid:

- Beef
- Buffalo
- Chicken (dark meat)
- Lamb
- Pork

Oils

Kaphas are already oily and heavy in nature so they don't need much oil, although a little should still be incorporated in the Kapha diet. Choose light, unprocessed oils. Water-sautéing is also good idea for Kaphas.

Oils Kaphas should favor:

- Almond oil
- Extra-virgin olive oil (small amounts)

- Flaxseed oil
- Ghee

Oils Kaphas should avoid:

- Canola oil
- Safflower oil

- Soy oil

Sweeteners

Kaphas should steer clear of sweets because they make them heavier and denser. The only sweetener Ayurveda recommends for Kaphas is raw honey in small amounts.

However, today we have sweeteners that don't make an impact on blood sugar levels, such as monk fruit sweetener, stevia, and birchwood xylitol, which can be incorporated in a Kapha diet to satisfy a sweet tooth without attributing to weight gain. I added an asterisk (*) to the new sweetener alternatives that did not exist in Ayurvedic times so you can differentiate.

Sweeteners Kaphas should favor:

- Birchwood xylitol*
- Honey (raw)

- Monk fruit sweetener*
- Stevia (liquid, organic)*

Sweeteners Kaphas should avoid:

- Artificial sweeteners
- Barley malt
- Date sugar
- Fructose

- Honey (cooked, heated, or processed)
- Maple syrup
- White sugar

AYURVEDIC ALERT

Look out for sneaky sugar hidden in savory foods such as sauces, dressings, and even ketchup. You'd be surprised by how much sugar you are unknowingly consuming in your everyday meals thanks to these products. Try to make your own food from scratch to avoid these sneaky sugar sources.

Spices

Spices are especially medicinal for Kaphas because they stimulate the digestive fire and speed up metabolisms. All spices are wonderful for Kaphas, with the exception of excess salt. Ginger, cinnamon, coriander, chili powder, and cayenne are particularly healing.

Spices Kaphas should favor:

- Ajwan
- Anise
- Asafoetida
- Basil
- Bay leaf
- Black pepper
- Cardamom
- Cayenne
- Cinnamon
- Cloves
- Coriander
- Cumin

- Fennel
- Fenugreek
- Garlic
- Ginger
- Mint
- Mustard seeds
- Nutmeg
- Oregano
- Paprika
- Rosemary
- Saffron
- Turmeric

Spices Kaphas should minimize:

- Excess salt

Sample Kapha Recipe

Kapha is a cold and heavy energy, therefore does best with lightly spiced, warm meals. They often have sluggish digestive fires, which can get a little boost with pungent tastes, stimulating spices, and easy-to-digest soups.

Spiced Lentil and Vegetable Soup

While Pittas should avoid excess spices, garlic and onions, Kaphas should run towards them. One of my favorite ways of getting in medicinal spices is through this Spiced Lentil and Vegetable Soup. The mustard seeds, ginger and cayenne stimulate Kaphas' slow metabolisms and the celery, carrots and tomatoes fill them up while keeping them light. This makes a perfect dinner for a Kapha type to help nourish them off to sleep.

1 TB. extra virgin olive oil or ghee

1 TB. brown mustard seeds (optional)

1 medium yellow onion, chopped

2 cloves garlic, minced

3 or 4 small peeled carrots, sliced

3 large ribs celery, sliced

1 cup tomatoes, chopped

1 cup brown lentils

1 TB. fresh ginger, grated

1 tsp. cumin

1 tsp. dried oregano

$1/4$ tsp. cayenne (or more to taste)

Ground black pepper

1 tsp. salt

4 cups water or low-sodium vegetable broth

1. In large pot over medium heat, heat olive oil or ghee and add mustard seeds (if using). Toast for 1 to 2 minutes or until you hear a popping sound, which means they are activated. Add yellow onion and garlic, sautéing for 3 minutes or until golden brown.

2. Add carrots, celery, and tomatoes to the pot, and sauté for 5 minutes.

3. Add brown lentils, ginger, cumin, oregano, cayenne, black pepper, sea salt, and water or low-sodium vegetable broth. Increase heat to medium-high, and bring to a boil.

4. Reduce heat to medium-low, cover, and simmer for 30 minutes or until lentils are tender.

5. Serve warm in a bowl. Top with a squeeze of lemon or lime or fresh herbs if you like.

WISDOM OF THE AGES

Ayurveda recommends toasting mustard seeds to impart the pungent taste. They have warming qualities and are great for the digestive system, making them especially beneficial for Kaphas and Vatas. When you hear the popping sound, that means they are activated and ready to use.

The recipes in this chapter offer just a sampling of the many wonderful dishes you can eat on an Ayurvedic diet. I share lots more in Part 4.

The Least You Need to Know

- Your digestion is referred to as your digestive fire, or agni. You want to eat foods that are easiest for your body to break down, absorb, and assimilate according to your Doshic constitution.

- Vatas can eat all sweet fruits, cooked vegetables, warming grains, few legumes, most organic dairy, all nuts and seeds, moist animal products, warming oils, most natural sweeteners, and a rich array of spices. They should stay away from dry or sour fruits, raw vegetables, cooling grains, and difficult-to-digest legumes.

- Pittas can eat all sweet fruits, most vegetables with the exception of nightshades, cooling grains, all legumes, some organic dairy, few nuts, all seeds, dry animal products, cooling oils, some natural sweeteners, and spices that aren't too hot. They should stay away from citrus fruit, nightshades, excess garlic and onions, warming grains, and excess nuts.

- Kaphas can eat less-sweet fruit, most vegetables, light grains, all legumes, no dairy, no nuts, all seeds, dry and light animal products, light oils, few natural sweeteners, and all spices. They should stay away from sweet fruit, raw vegetables, heavy grains, all dairy, and nuts.

CHAPTER 7

Nature Versus Imbalance

Now that you have an idea of what your Dosha is, I'm going to make things a tad more confusing, but bear with me. The Dosha you have today may be different from the one you were born with. Crazy, I know, but it is actually quite intuitive once you get the hang of it.

You have something called your *Prakriti,* which is your natural Doshic constitution given at the moment of birth. This includes your skin color, height, hair color, and other predetermined characteristics. Then you have your *Vikruti,* which is the Doshic constitution you have today. This is who you are due to your diet and lifestyle choices, such as when you gain or lose weight. Your Vikruti is affected by a host of factors, including your environment, age, stress level, and the amount of exercise you get.

In this chapter, I explain the difference between your Prakriti and Vikruti and how you can assess your own.

In This Chapter

- The difference between the Dosha you were born with and the one you have today
- Assessing your Prakriti and Vikruti
- The causes of each Dosha's imbalance
- Understanding your imbalances

Prakriti

While reading the descriptions of the Doshas in Chapters 4 and 5, you might have found that you related to all of them at different points in your life. Maybe in your 20s you were totally Pitta, and now you feel completely Kapha. That's normal. You have all the Doshas within you in varying amounts, and they change throughout your life. But how do you know what you truly are and what's just temporary? By addressing the difference between your Prakriti and your Vikruti.

Your Prakriti is who you are. Some of us are naturally born lanky, and others of us are bigger boned. These characteristics are in your DNA. You can lose or gain weight, but you cannot change your genetic makeup. I was born as a brown-eyed, round-faced, small-boned brunette of medium height. There is no way I'm going to end up as a blue-eyed, angular-faced, big-boned blonde who is 6 feet tall. It's just not in the cards for me.

However, I can change some things. Maybe I become a body builder or let myself go and gain 50 pounds. But it isn't who I am. It's just my Vikruti, my current Doshic state. Your Vikruti shows you where your imbalances are. The secret to health is coming back to your natural Doshic constitution, your Prakriti.

> **DEFINITION**
>
> The Doshic constitution you were born with is called your **Prakriti,** and it was decided for you at the moment of conception. The Doshic constitution you have today is your **Vikruti** and illustrates your imbalances. The key to health is making your Vikruti come back to your Prakriti.

Your Prakriti isn't just one Dosha but a unique combination of the three. For example, my Prakriti is primarily Kapha, secondarily Vata, and lastly Pitta. However, my Vikruti today is primarily Vata, secondarily Kapha, and lastly Pitta. I am now more Vata than I am Kapha, although I was born with Kapha traits. I have to be careful of my Vata falling off balance because I am not naturally a Vata type. I became this way through diet and exercise. However, whenever I take Dosha quizzes, my results indicate that I am a Vata because that's what my highest Dosha is today. Let's discover yours.

The Dosha You Were Born With

At the moment of conception, your entire genetic makeup was formulated. The color of your hair and skin, your height, your personal characteristics, and even the diseases you are prone to were all picked for you. This is your Prakriti. It's essentially the deck of cards you were handed at birth, as unique as your fingerprint.

No matter what you eat or do, these are things you cannot change, such as your bone structure, the areas you gain fat, or how your skin reacts in the sun. Your Prakriti is what you are in your truest form. You may be able to hide or manipulate it, but it will always remain.

Your Vikruti, on the other hand, is the Doshic constitution you have today. In fact, most likely what you scored on the quiz in Chapter 4 is your Vikruti, not your Prakriti. Your Vikruti describes what your Doshic constitution is like at the present moment. It's related to your dietary and lifestyle choices, as well as environmental factors.

It's easy to confuse your Vikruti as your Prakriti, but they are not the same. To determine your Prakriti, you must think about what you were naturally like as a child and what you are like without any manipulation. That shows you how your body was designed and what it's disposed to. Then you can determine how your current habits and other lifestyle factors play a role in the way your body is today.

WISDOM OF THE AGES

The secret to health is having your Vikruti match your Prakriti. Your body naturally wants to maintain balance. When you stray from your natural rhythm, that's when things tend to go off balance.

To show you what these Doshas are like in action, let's go over three cases so you can see the difference between the Prakriti and Vikruti.

Case 1: Vata

Paul is a Vata Prakriti. He's always been a thin guy who had a hard time gaining weight. Now in college, he decides he is sick of being the lanky guy and wants to put on muscle and bulk up his physique. He starts lifting weights, eating lots of protein, and upping his calories. Unlike a Pitta Prakriti, he has a tough time gaining weight, let alone muscle, yet with persistence, he eventually succeeds. After a few months, you would never even guess he is a Vata. He's strong, built, and has the exact body type as a Pitta. He takes the Dosha quiz and assesses that he is a Pitta.

However, he begins experiencing Vata imbalances. He becomes constipated from eating all this meat his Pitta friends have no problem with due to their increased stomach acid. He often feels light-headed during his workouts and needs to sit down. He notices tremors in his muscles, too. All these are signs of Vata. Although Paul may look and feel like a Pitta, he remains a Vata Prakriti. His natural Vata characteristics came out because that is what he was born with. To remain balanced, he must continue pacifying his Vata.

Case 2: Pitta

Kathy is a Pitta Prakriti. She was always an athletic child with a fast metabolism and strong digestion. She remained active throughout her 20s and had a muscular figure. However, now, in her 30s, she is going through a rough patch in her life and lets herself go. She begins emotionally eating and ceases all physical activity. She starts gaining weight, which continues to accumulate over the years. She's now 50 pounds overweight and huffs and puffs just going up the stairs. She loses interest in any type of movement or group activity and prefers to be on the couch watching television. She takes the Dosha quiz and sees that she is a Kapha—overweight, sedentary, heavy, and depressed.

However, her Prakriti is not a Kapha. She was never overweight growing up and isn't naturally bigger-boned or reclusive. She is overweight only because of her sugar-laden diet, lack of movement, and situational sadness. Her Vikruti is Kapha, which is why she is experiencing all the side effects, but her Prakriti remains Pitta. If she just removes the heavy, fried, and sugary foods from her diet; adds more spices to her meals; and becomes more active to boost her Pitta, the weight will slip off easily. Unlike someone who was born Kapha and naturally bigger-boned, this weight is not hers to hold. It is caused from an imbalance.

Case 3: Kapha

Lauren is a Kapha Prakriti. She always has been curvy-figured and as long as she can remember, she's had trouble with her weight. She feels like she was born on a diet, none of which ever work for very long. However, she decides that enough is enough and she will do whatever it takes to lose weight. She goes on a detox diet, eating only raw vegetables, seeds, and a few other safety foods. Even when she is hungry, she denies her body of food to stick to her "diet." Eventually, she loses all the weight she wanted to lose.

However, it doesn't really feel like a celebration. She is exhausted and feels cold all the time. After a while, she stops menstruating, her hair begins to shed, and her skin loses the vibrant glow it once had. She doesn't understand how some people can naturally be so thin while her body is literally shutting down to maintain her "goal weight."

She takes the Dosha quiz and gets the result for Vata—cold, underweight, thin hair, dry skin. However, she isn't a Vata Prakriti. She has to starve herself to sustain this figure. She is experiencing Vata imbalances because her Vikruti is Vata but her Prakriti remains Kapha. The healthiest weight for her is different from her goal weight. It's the weight her body needs to be at to maintain balance. By denying her natural body type, she is only hurting herself.

Assessing Your Natural Tendencies

Now that you see what these cases are like, I want you to think about your own and where you stand. Look back at pictures from your childhood. What did you look like? Were you a scrawny kid? A natural athlete? A chubby little one? How and when did that change? Was it natural or manipulated? Is your body healthy at your current weight?

Your Shifting Vikruti

The Doshas are fluid, dynamic, and ever-moving, like the seasons. Similarly, your Vikruti shifts over the course of the year and throughout your life. In this section, I discuss factors that can affect your Vikruti, including your lifestyle, environment, and diet. That way, you will know what might be causing your current Doshic imbalance. Remember, for your health, you must make an effort to rebalance your Vikruti to match your Prakriti.

> **WISDOM OF THE AGES**
>
> Your Vikruti, the Doshic constitution you have today, is what causes imbalances. The negative symptoms you experience, from bloating to insomnia, are related to your Vikruti. To regain health, you must rebalance your Vikruti to match your Prakriti.

You can have imbalances of any of the Doshas, even if they are not your predominant one. For example, in cold, dry weather, you are at risk of Vata imbalances. In cold, wet weather, you are more likely to face Kapha imbalances. In hot, humid weather, you are more likely to face Pitta imbalances. Other factors such as your stress levels and daily habits also affect your Vikruti.

Let's look at some common causes of imbalances related to each Dosha so you can see them in yourself.

Causes of Vata Imbalance

A Vata imbalance can be caused by cold and dry weather, undereating or going long times without food, eating lots of raw or cold foods, excess cardio, travel, or doing too many things at once.

Vata is a cold and dry energy, so being in such a climate causes your Vata to fall off balance. This is why you tend to experience many of the Vata side effects in the autumn.

Vata is a naturally light energy that needs to be balanced with grounding. When you undereat or fast, you don't get the calories you need to function. This makes your body go into stress mode as it tries to find energy to sustain itself. This also causes a Vata imbalance.

Some people, like Vata Prakritis, are thin by nature despite eating abundantly, but others force their bodies into a smaller size by undereating, in part because of the media's portrayal of thin, Vata bodies as the most desirable. Many women have to restrict their diets to lose weight, but this also cuts in to their nutritional intake, making them malnourished. Hair loss, chills, dry skin, and amenorrhea (the loss of a menstrual cycle for more than 3 months) all have become increasingly common due to this widespread Vata imbalance. Malnourishment puts women at risk for infertility, anemia, osteoporosis, and other Vata-related side effects.

Travel and lack of routine can cause a Vata imbalance. When you fly, your body takes on airy qualities, increasing your Vata energy. Dry skin, lips, and hair; insomnia; and jet-lag are all common with and after travel. This is why it's important to particularly pacify your Vata while you're on the go. We spend more and more time every day in transit, putting our bodies in a chronic, subtle state of stress.

With busier, more hectic lives, people have less time to sit down and eat warm, cooked meals. Throughout history around the world, people traditionally ate three home-cooked meals a day. Today, most of us are lucky to get one. We have become a snack culture, eating frequently but never truly enjoying a meal. Most snack foods are cold, dry, and rough—think granola bars, popcorn, or chips—which increase Vata energy. It's important to incorporate warm, grounding, cooked foods in your diet, whether you're a Vata type or not, because cooked foods are easiest for your body to digest and absorb.

As we spend more time at desk jobs and sitting in transit, we often look for the most intense exercise as possible to "make up" for those sedentary hours. Fast-paced cardio classes have become increasingly popular to burn the largest amount of calories in the shortest amount of time. From an Ayurvedic perspective, however, this can be extremely harmful.

Excess cardio increases your Vata energy because Vata is related to movement energy. It's not healthy for your body to go from sitting all day to huffing and out of breath. Instead, it's much more effective to move and walk regularly throughout the day, without burning yourself out. If you overrun your body, you'll feel Vata side effects, including restlessness, aching joints, insomnia, muscle tremors, or injury. It's better to exercise slowly but deliberately to keep your body in check.

What Happens When Your Vata Is Excess?

When your Vata is excess, you start feeling Vata imbalances, including bloating; gas; constipation; cramping; cold body temperature; hair loss; dry eyes, skin, mouth, nose, and hair; irregular or missed periods; back pain; short-term memory loss; forgetfulness; insomnia; restlessness; and/or anxiety.

You might not experience all these imbalances, but the more imbalanced your Vata becomes, the more they will manifest. This is why it's important to pacify your Vata before the problems pile on.

Causes of Pitta Imbalance

A Pitta imbalance can be caused by hot weather, stress, caffeine, spicy food, excess exercise and especially strength training, and a competitive environment.

> **WISDOM OF THE AGES**
>
> Have you ever noticed you felt in a bad mood when the air-conditioning wasn't working? That's because your Pitta was off balance. Hot weather causes your body to overheat, cranking up your internal fire until you can't take it. Many people become more irritable in hot weather for this very reason.

It's especially important for Pitta types to stay out of direct sunlight in the middle of the day, when the sun is highest, and exercise either early in the morning or in the afternoon, when the sun is lower in the sky. Exercising while overheated causes a severe Pitta imbalance because exercise already heats the body.

Stress definitely causes a Pitta imbalance. When you have a million things to do, you become overwhelmed and sometimes snap. This is why it's important to always take a break, even if you aren't a Pitta, to cool down stored-up tension. Stress creates heat in the system, which turns into acne, acidity, and a whole host of other Pitta imbalances you don't want to suffer from.

Caffeine triggers Pitta because it's a stimulant … and that's why Pittas love it, even though it's the last thing they need. Stimulants make your blood pump faster, exciting your inner Pitta to achieve and do more. Caffeine feeds the fire, but eventually that fire goes out, making you feel even worse … and crave more caffeine. People often become addicted to caffeine because of the Pitta rush it provides, especially Pitta types who are addicted to performance. Caffeine is extremely acidic and causes further heartburn, irritation, acne, and ulcers in a Pittas' already acidic body.

What Happens When Your Pitta Is Excess?

When your Pitta is excess, you'll start feeling Pitta imbalance symptoms, including hyperacidity, excess sweating, foul-smelling odor, overheating, premature gray hair and balding, oily skin, acne, rosacea, indigestion, impatience, anger, and/or aggression.

You might not experience all these things, but the more imbalanced your Pitta becomes, the more these symptoms will manifest, which is why it's important to prevent and pacify them.

Causes of Kapha Imbalance

A Kapha imbalance can be caused by cold, rainy, or snowy weather; overeating; eating too many sweet, rich, or fatty foods; a sedentary lifestyle; under exercising; and depression.

Have you ever felt like staying in bed all day, week, or even month? Have you gone through a period of time when you just feel too exhausted for life? Have you ever dealt with your emotions by stuffing yourself with food? These are times when your Kapha is out of balance.

Kapha is a heavy and dense energy and makes you feel likewise. It can be brought on by cold, wet weather, which is why many of us gain weight during the winter. Leading a sedentary life-style and sitting for long periods of time further heightens the imbalance. Additionally, when you stay in your comfort zone, you lose the motivation to try new things, contributing more to the imbalance.

> **WISDOM OF THE AGES**
>
> The less you move your body, the less it wants to move. You may have noticed how easily you fall off the bandwagon after several weeks without exercise. After a hiatus, every bit of movement becomes incredibly difficult because your Kapha is heightened.

We live in a society in which we're forced to sit many hours a day for work and school, so it's important to work to keep your Kapha from creeping up, causing you to become lazy and inactive, even during your off hours. Make a point to move around during the day, even if it's to go for a brisk walk or do a few jumping jacks every 30 minutes to get your heart rate going and keep you in fat-burning mode. Working at a standing desk can help you remain active while you work.

Eating too many sweet, rich, or fatty foods also increase your Kapha levels. Sweet foods, including breads and pastas, make you feel more lethargic and cause your blood sugar levels to rapidly increase, which means weight gain. Fatty foods are difficult for your body to digest and slow down your metabolic rate. Rich foods are dense in calories and cause heaviness in your body and your mind. It's crucial for Kaphas to consume a light, portion-controlled diet with bitter and well-spiced foods as well as lead active lifestyles.

What Happens When Your Kapha Is Excess?

When your Kapha is excess, you'll start feeling Kapha imbalance symptoms, including weight-gain, lethargy, diabetes, water retention, mucus, slow digestion and metabolism, cold body temperature, clammy hands, sadness, emotional eating and/or depression.

You might not experience all these symptoms, but the more imbalanced your Kapha becomes, the more these symptoms will manifest, which is why it's important to prevent and pacify them.

Knowing Your Imbalances

It's normal to experience imbalances of all three Doshas. There may have been a time you were overweight, causing a Kapha imbalance. You may have undergone a period of stress, attributing to a Pitta imbalance. Or maybe you got burnt out and became fatigued, leading to a Vata imbalance. The Doshas are ever-flowing energies that cause your Vikruti to change throughout your life.

Learn the difference between your Prakriti and Vikruti so you can properly treat your body. When following Ayurvedic guidelines, always choose the suggestions for the Dosha that's off balance, your Vikruti. This pacifies the Dosha that's off balance so you can revert to your Prakriti. For example, if your Kapha is off balance, causing you to become heavy and lethargic, follow a Kapha-pacifying diet. If your Vata is out of balance, causing you to be become malnourished and constipated, follow a Vata-pacifying diet. If your Pitta is not in check, causing you to experience heartburn and loose stools, follow a Pitta-pacifying diet.

You still want to keep your Prakriti in mind, however, and check back in with your body often. Follow the Vikruti-pacifying guidelines until you no longer suffer from that imbalance and then gradually adjust your diet so you can maintain your own unique version of balance.

So many things can attribute to a Dosha imbalance, and knowing them can help you avoid a lifetime of disease. You have a great deal of control over your well-being. All it takes is awareness and responsibility.

The Least You Need to Know

- The Doshic constitution you were born with is called your Prakriti; the one you have today is your Vikruti.
- You are not just one Dosha but a combination of all three, and that combination may change throughout your life.
- Certain dietary and lifestyle decisions, such as eating, exercising, or sleeping too much, cause an imbalance in your Vikruti.
- The secret to health is making your Vikruti match your Prakriti.

8

Lifestyle Practices for Each Dosha

I've talked a lot about diet to balance the Doshas, but lifestyle is equally as important. Even if you eat the right foods, if you continue to lead a lifestyle that contrasts with what your Doshic needs are, you are going to remain imbalanced.

In this chapter, I share some lifestyle recommendations for each Dosha. I also give you a specific life lesson each Dosha has to work on. Finally, I offer the best yoga practices and meditation methods for each Dosha so you know how to bring yours back into balance, both mentally and physically.

In This Chapter

- Recommended lifestyle tips for each Dosha
- Key lessons for each Dosha to work on
- Optimal yoga practices for every Dosha
- The best ways for each Dosha to meditate

Vata Practices

Vatas can be a bit all over the place—blame it on the excess wind. The air and ether (space) energy within Vatas makes them particularly flighty, overwhelmed, and scattered. This is why it's important for Vatas to establish a grounding practice that settles their irregular appetite, their digestive system, and even their moods. The one lesson Vatas really need to work on is grounding.

By following these practices, you Vatas can find much more peace and harmony in your day-to-day life. You'll be less affected by stress and anxiety and become much stronger in your will. Grounding provides the structure you need to see tasks through, and you'll finally be able to finish all those genius projects you started but haven't yet gotten around to completing.

Routine provides the awareness to know what's coming next, which prepares your mind and body for eating, sleeping, digesting, etc. Your mind and body are much more effective at what they do when you know what you're going to throw at them, and these practices will help build that intuitive awareness.

Establish a Routine

Having a routine does not come naturally for those with a Vata mind. You prefer to take things as they come, and one day may look completely different from the next. To you, routines feel like an invasion of your personal freedom. You'd much rather feel out things.

Now there's nothing wrong with spontaneity, and some people thrive in less-structured schedules. However, you do need some sort of consistency in your day-to-day life. That doesn't mean you repeat the same tasks in the same place every day, but you do need to have some sort of daily routine, including self-care and timing your meals, so your body knows what to expect. You function best when you have a routine because your body is prepared to digest, relax, sleep, etc.

Vatas highly benefit from establishing a daily routine, or dinacharya. Here's an example of a great daily routine for Vatas:

> Wake up around the same time each day (ideally at dawn).
>
> Practice morning routine (which I discuss more in Chapter 10): eliminate, brush teeth, scrape tongue, wash face, oil pull with sesame oil.
>
> Drink a hot cup of warming tea, such as ginger, and meditate.
>
> Eat a warm breakfast, such as cooked grains with almond milk and cinnamon.
>
> Begin your day in a peaceful manner.

Eat lunch around the same time every day. Do not snack randomly throughout the day but just have one in the afternoon, if you're hungry.

Exercise in the afternoon when your energy levels are up.

Eat an early, easy-to-digest dinner like vegetable stew.

Enjoy a nightly warm tonic like turmeric golden mylk, an ancient plant-based Ayurvedic elixir, comprised of turmeric seeped in nondairy milk.

Oil your body with sesame oil, and turn off all technology.

Get to sleep soundly by 10 P.M.

When you have a different routine every day, your body doesn't know what to anticipate. A routine allows your body to expect certain things at certain times—when you're going to rise, eat, exercise, sleep, and various other functions—so it can prepare itself for that role. If one day you eat at 9 P.M. and the next day you're in bed at that time, your body will be confused because it won't know what to prepare for. Routines do not take away from your freedom but actually give you more of it. You are free when you are healthy, which is why a consistent routine is important, especially for Vatas.

Slow It Down

Vatas tend to go at the speed of light, which causes them to go into overdrive and burn out. The real medicine for Vatas is to slow down. When you go through life slowly, you become more deliberate in your actions and gain awareness. This awareness brings more years to your life and life to your years.

WISDOM OF THE AGES

In yogic tradition, it's believed you only have a certain amount of breaths in your lifetime. If you breathe too fast, you'll move through them quickly and have a shorter lifespan. Take things slow, and breathe deeply and meaningfully as if you were sucking in more life with each breath.

Vatas should practice doing just one task at a time to achieve mindfulness. Rather than multitasking, you should see one undertaking through before beginning the next. It's especially crucial that you slow down and be mindful while you're eating because Vatas often eat standing up, while talking, or even when driving. This prevents your digestive system from functioning properly because your body doesn't know whether it should be focusing on eating or the other activity simultaneously going on.

Slow down. Breathe. Tune in. Take your time. Don't stress about how many things you have to do. You are a human *being,* not a human *doing.* Make your first task being so you better achieve the doing.

Yoga Practice

Yoga is a beneficial way for you to use your Vata body in a way that's conductive, not destructive. Vatas often have surges of energy they need to release, which causes them to go a million miles an hour and then crash. Yoga teaches awareness and taking things slow—two lessons Vatas dearly need to learn.

> **AYURVEDIC ALERT**
>
> Vatas also frequently suffer from skeletal issues, such as back pain and popping joints. If untreated, this can turn into arthritis, osteoporosis, and injury. Yoga can teach you alignment and help you strengthen loose joints.

Not all yoga practices are created equally. Vatas must practice grounding, structured, and strength-building yoga postures to counterbalance their flighty, irregular, and highly flexible minds and bodies. Vatas often have no problem winding their way through an active Vinyasa yoga class or stretching into a deep split. However, if they do not build the strength to match that flexibility and movement, they are at risk of getting hurt. Vatas also are often born with abnormalities, causing them to suffer from poor balance. They must take extra precaution to work on alignment and be sure the left and right sides of their bodies are proportioned.

Now let's take a look at some recommended yoga poses for Vatas.

Sun salutation: *surya namaskar,* or the sun salutation, is the cornerstone of any dynamic yoga practice. It is considered the "crest jewel of yoga" because of its benefits for the mind, body, and spirit.

The sun salutation is a series of postures that open every channel of your body, heat your internal fire, and prepare your muscles for practice. The sequence is recommended for all Doshas; however, you Vatas should particularly pay attention to your alignment to ensure you're reaping the benefits of the practice, staying in your range of mobility, and keeping your joints safe. Time your breath with each pose to truly get the best of the practice.

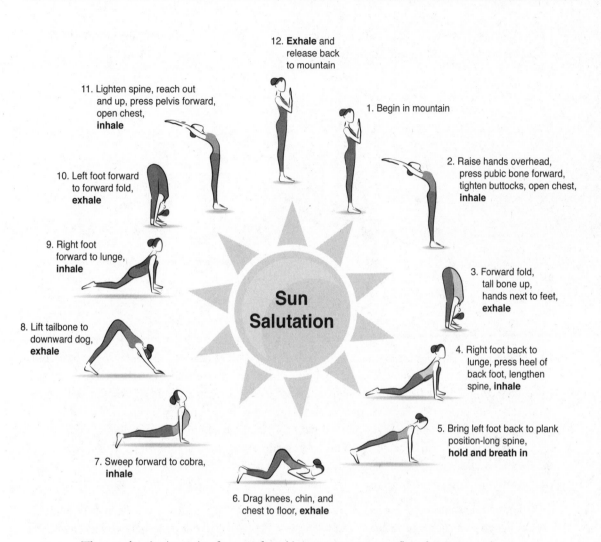

12. **Exhale** and release back to mountain

11. Lighten spine, reach out and up, press pelvis forward, open chest, **inhale**

10. Left foot forward to forward fold, **exhale**

9. Right foot forward to lunge, **inhale**

8. Lift tailbone to downward dog, **exhale**

7. Sweep forward to cobra, **inhale**

6. Drag knees, chin, and chest to floor, **exhale**

1. Begin in mountain

2. Raise hands overhead, press pubic bone forward, tighten buttocks, open chest, **inhale**

3. Forward fold, tall bone up, hands next to feet, **exhale**

4. Right foot back to lunge, press heel of back foot, lengthen spine, **inhale**

5. Bring left foot back to plank position-long spine, **hold and breath in**

Sun Salutation

The sun salutation is a series of poses performed in a sequence to create a flow of movement, each pose coordinating with your breath. As a rule of thumb, inhale to extend and exhale to bend.

Warrior pose: The warrior pose II, *virabhadrasana* II, builds strength, vitality, and grounding in the body. You not only use your leg muscles to support yourself but also your spine to keep your body upright and your arms and chest to remain open. Although this pose may appear like you're just standing there, it's actually extremely difficult when done the right way. With warrior pose II, you are teaching your body to be rooted and supported, while still open and expansive.

Oftentimes in weight training, it's easy to tense your muscles in order to be strong. The warrior pose II gives you the benefits of a muscular workout without even needing to move. It is through stillness that you cultivate true strength. This is particularly difficult for Vatas, who always feel the need to move.

Hold warrior II pose for 1 to 3 minutes, getting deeper as the time goes on. Practicing this pose cultivates true grounding and strength, bringing out the powerful warrior within you.

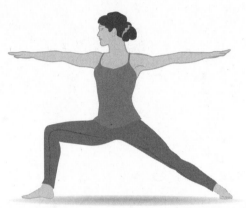

Warrior II is a standing pose that enhances strength, stability and concentration, commemorating the Hindu mythological warrior Virabhadra, an incarnation of the god Shiva.

Dancer's pose: The dancer's pose, *natarajasana,* is especially beneficial for Vatas for two reasons. First, as you can see, it requires serious balance. Vatas' minds are often scattered all over the place, but to practice this pose, you must cultivate awareness. One unrelated thought, and you'll fall out of the pose. This is particularly helpful during times of anxiety when your mind is racing. Instead of becoming overwhelmed with the situation, simply practice dancer's pose. It will force your mind to become centered, and the more balanced you become, the more you can expand your body. Vatas also are prone to bone abnormalities and muscular weakness and especially need to work on balance to prevent injury.

The second reason this pose is especially effective for Vatas is because it is known as the wind-relieving pose. That means what it sounds like—it allows your body to expel extra gas from your colon. Vatas particularly have an issue with gas accumulation, so this pose can help naturally release any air bubbles that may have been collecting in the colon. Don't be nervous about doing this pose in public. After some repetition, you will no longer pass any gas with this pose, making it safe to practice in any yoga class.

> **WISDOM OF THE AGES**
>
> Yoga is not about how high you can hold up your leg or deep you can get your squat. It is about connection with the breath and staying true to your own practice, wherever that is today.

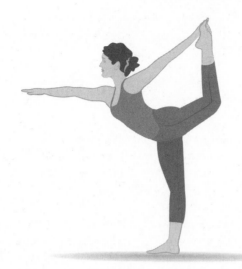

"Nata" means dancer while "raja": means king and "asana" means pose in Sanskrit. Natarajasana is the "lord of the dance" pose and requires full-body strength, flexibility and focus.

Meditation Tips

If you're like most Vatas, you have a tough time with meditation because while you're trying to quiet and center yourself, suddenly your to-do list comes to mind, taking you elsewhere. Because it's not natural for you, you should practice so you're more effective at it and receptive to it.

Vatas waste a lot of time worrying about their worries. With meditation, you can come into center and gain the mental strength you need to tackle your to-do list, one task at a time, without becoming overwhelmed by its enormity.

Find a comfortable way to meditate. Because many Vatas have skeletal issues, sitting in cross-legged position on the floor with no back support can be painful, taking you out of your zone. If your body is in pain, you can't focus on transcending into your highest self—all you can think about is that pain! Vatas really can benefit from a meditation chair, a padded chair placed on the floor with a supported back. That way, you can focus on your growing consciousness, not the growing tension in your back.

Vatas particularly need something to focus on during meditation or their minds will race, so set a focus to your meditation with a mantra or affirmation. We all have something we need to work on—it could be garnering more inner peace or abundance. Meditation is the perfect time to channel this by repeating it in your mind or aloud. Your thoughts turn into your reality, and by chanting your desires, they're more likely to manifest.

Some people really benefit from chanting in Sanskrit, while others love to repeat positive affirmations in their native language. Ayurveda recommends chanting in Sanskrit because it is considered a divine language. Sanskrit is the first-ever recorded language of mankind, and many Hindus believe it is the "language of the gods." Even though Hindi is now the spoken language of India, prayers are still chanted in Sanskrit.

> **WISDOM OF THE AGES**
>
> The Sanskrit language is especially powerful because each word was formulated to carry the specific vibration of its meaning. Linguists call it the perfect language because its grammar and intonation are so well thought out. In fact, the word *Sanskrit* itself actually means "well or completely formed." Each word was carefully selected for its vibration.

If you aren't sure what the "vibration" of a word means, just think about music. Every sound has a vibration, evoking a feeling within you. Similarly, the words we speak also have some sort of vibration. It's just like how an animal can pick up when you are speaking kind words or mean words, regardless of whether they actually understand what you're saying. It's the vibration your tone carries that they decipher. Sanskrit words were carefully created with attention to each letter's sound. Words in most other languages were just chosen, not based on their energetic effects, but on their derivative.

As the common phrase goes, "Sticks and stones may break my bones, but words can never hurt me." Sanskrit, on the other hand, would say, "Sticks and stones may break my bones, but words will truly heal me." This is why Sanskrit chanting is so popular around the world. The phrases chanted are called *mantras.* Mantras cannot be translated because translation alters the sound and they no longer hold the same power.

> **WISDOM OF THE AGES**
>
> When you enunciate a mantra, your tongue taps certain points of the roof of your mouth, sending signals to your hypothalamus, which regulates the chemical activity of your brain and whole body. By repeating the mantra, these sound patterns become inscribed in your brain and you wake up your dormant, unconscious mind. As you repeat the mantra, you get lost in its echo and your sense of ego temporarily fades. Your sounds carry electromagnetic vibrations and reflect your thoughts, and by elevating your vibrations by repeating sacred Sanskrit chants or positive affirmations, you elevate your thoughts. Mantras enhance your mood, intuition, awareness, compassion, and even immunity. Through mantra, you realize your own inner power and who you truly are.

You don't have to understand the meaning of a word to chant it as a mantra. In fact, mantras on their own do not have meaning. The power is not in the words but in the sound vibrations they carry. Whether you choose to chant in Sanskrit, English, or any other language is your choice. All that matters is it has resonance for you.

Pitta Practices

Pittas are sharp, determined, and fiery individuals who push their minds—and bodies—to the limit. They are go-getters who know what they want and will work at any lengths to achieve it. They are naturally very organized and thrive in structure. Unlike Vatas, they become extremely stressed if they don't know what's going to happen next and enjoy having a schedule to go by. You might see a Pitta have a color-coded calendar organized by each type of appointment, and their schedule is filled months in advance.

Routine and structure are great, but it's important Pittas aren't run by them. Pittas benefit from allowing more flow and spontaneity in their lives. Sometimes they have to sit back and trust that everything is going to work out, even if they don't hold the reins of control.

Pittas must work on chilling out, remaining mindful, and keeping their cool under all the pressure they find themselves. Their yoga and meditation practices should reflect that as well. A Vata's mantra is to ground down, and a Pitta's is to chill out.

Chill Out

I mean "chill out" not just figuratively but also literally. Pittas must work on keeping all things chill—mind, body, and spirit. When too much tension builds in the body, you experience heat. That heat accumulates and has nowhere to go. This causes acne, acidity, and even heart attacks and strokes in later years.

Many of us experience this pent-up heat on an everyday basis. Bursts of anger, impatience, or road rage are prime examples. You may have felt a sudden rush of tension overcoming your body that unexpectedly erupted as a rude comment or harsh tone you didn't really mean. You might not have even known that rage existed within you. It's stored heat.

It's healthy to release stored anger, but you must do it in a constructive and controlled fashion. You can exercise to release it, dance it out, or yell into nature to prevent yourself from snapping at another person. Ayurveda believes the best way to balance your anger is to cool it down. Rather than giving in to or fueling it, you must acknowledge its root source and counterbalance it with calming activities like yoga, tai chi, and meditation.

Pittas must learn that self-care and rest are just as important as productivity. They often struggle with work-life balance, so they need to set aside some time in their routine to rest. This does not mean lounging in front of the TV but rather sitting still under a tree, spending time with family, reading a book, playing with an animal, or taking a walk in nature.

Pittas are especially cooled down by the colors green and blue and should spend time near trees or water. Try taking a weekend trip to a nearby beach, lake, or forest. Pittas tend to spend a lot of time in front of the computer, and their eyes could really benefit from the break.

Practice Mindfulness

Pittas' minds are often full, but they are not mindful. To be mindful, one must be present in the moment. That means putting away your phone, not thinking about your next meeting, or sending emails while eating dinner.

Whatever you do, be completely there. When you're at work, be totally there (which Pittas have no problem with). But when you're with your family, be wholly present there. Don't waste your precious time with your loved ones worrying about work or planning tomorrow's work presentation. Pittas love their friends and family but sometimes have a tough time showing it. By being mindful, you'll be able to show them they are fully worthy of your time, presence, and love, which are one in the same.

Mindfulness is the key to mastering mind-full-ness. Your career, personal relations, digestion, and health will thrive if you are able to cultivate mindfulness in everything you do.

Stay Cool

This is the physical part of "chilling out" I was referring to. Pittas need to stay cool because their bodies are so hot. That means avoiding time in the direct sunlight, especially midday when the sun is highest in the sky. Instead, seek shadier spots and indoor activities to keep your body temperature stable.

Pittas become extremely irritable in the heat, which is why they are the type of people who always need air-conditioning. They should wear airy clothes, such as organic cotton, and stay away from nylon and polyester. They also should avoid exercising in the heat because it will make them feel nauseated afterward. The best time for them to exercise is in the morning before the sun gets too hot.

Here's an example of a great daily routine for Pittas:

Wake up around the same time each day (ideally right before dawn).

Practice morning routine: eliminate, brush teeth, scrape tongue, wash face, oil pull with coconut oil.

Drink a warm cup of cooling tea, such as coriander, and meditate.

Practice yoga, tai chi, Pilates, or another calming exercise.

Eat your breakfast, preferably warm.

Stay mindful with all your tasks, and keep your stress levels low.

Make lunch your biggest meal of the day. If you get hungry again in the afternoon, have a snack.

Take a walk outside and cool off your body.

Enjoy an early, easily digested dinner like steamed vegetables and beans.

Sip a nightly warm tonic, oil your body with sesame or coconut oil, and turn off all technology

Get to sleep soundly by 10 P.M., before you get your second wind of energy.

Yoga Practice

Pittas are often the ones in front of the class, secretly competing with each other for who can hold a handstand longer. However, that competitive energy is the exact opposite of what Pittas need. Focus on the more yin, meditative, restorative aspect of yoga to ease your already tense Pitta mind and body.

Yin yoga is the practice of holding a single stretch for several minutes, allowing your body to release into it. Vinyasa yoga classes take you through many moves within an hour, but yin yoga forces you to really sit in the pose and feel its effects on your body. This is much harder for Pitta types, who always feel the need to perform. They love holding planks and inversions but actually need more flexibility in their tight muscles. Pittas should focus on yoga that opens their hips, backs, shoulders, and legs.

Rag doll pose: The rag doll pose, or *uttanasana,* is a great release for the head, neck, and shoulders. By bending forward and allowing gravity do its work, you stretch your entire spinal cord.

To practice rag doll, simply bend at your hips, and with your hands, hold on to your elbows to allow your upper body to hang heavy. Slowly shift side to side to release the tension in both sides of your lower back. Gently bend your knees to feel the stretch more in your hips. Nod your head to release any tension in your neck. Let your back really sink into this pose, feeling its deep release.

This pose is great for times when tension has built up and you feel like you're about to burst. You can practice it any time of day, except an hour after a meal. Rag doll soothes the adrenals, relieves tension headaches, and gets blood flowing back to your brain, giving you a creative pick-me-up.

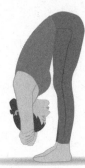

Rag doll isn't about how hard you can push but how much you can release. The more you allow
yourself to fall into this pose, the more beneficial it will be.

Reclining butterfly pose: This pose helps open tight hip muscles, where Pittas often store tension. It is believed that your hips are where you hold emotional pain. By opening your hips, unresolved emotions may come up. Instead of suppressing them, let them flow through you.

To practice reclining butterfly, or *supta baddha konasana,* simply lie down on your back, place the soles of your feet together, and feel the stretch in your inner hips. For a deeper stretch, gently press down on your inner thighs. I recommend practicing this pose in bed before you sleep each night. It's an easy pose to hold while you drift off to sleep. Remember to breathe deeply to allow your tight muscles to expand.

It is entirely normal to start crying during hip-opening poses. You may not even know why. It is just your body releasing any emotional traumas it may still be holding onto. Trust the process, and allow yourself to be vulnerable. This is especially difficult for Pittas, who need full control at all times. They often move past an issue without really mourning it or feeling its full pain or sadness. This causes the emotional pain to linger in the body, particularly in the psoas, a muscle that runs inside your hips. Open hips, open life. By loosening any stored negative emotions, you create space for new positive ones.

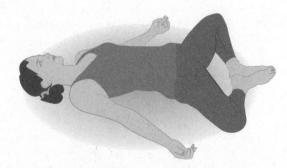

Give yourself a few minutes to really fall into this pose and allow the release of your hips. This pose is
best performed after a workout.

Child's pose: This is one of the most universally popular yoga poses because of its immense benefits and ease. Child's pose, also called *balasana*, soothes your overworked adrenals and signals to your nervous system to rest. It gives your body the same rested feeling as being back in your mother's womb, if you could remember what that felt like. It also stretches tight lower backs, which can tense up from hours of sitting. This is an easy pose to practice that requires no physical tension.

To get into child's pose, simply rest on your knees and sit back on your calves. Slowly bend forward and lower yourself so your upper body is lying over your thighs. Extend your arms forward, stretching your spine. It also feels really great to have someone push down on your lower back to really extend the stretch. Our kidneys are in our lower-back area and can get a really nice massage with this pose.

This is a really great pose to get into when the tension of the day is too high and you just need to unwind. It instantly alerts your body that it's safe to rest. I recommend keeping a yoga mat in your office so you have a clean place to do this pose because your face will be on the ground.

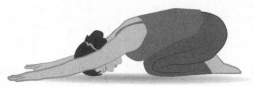

Child's pose is considered the resting pose in yoga and recommended between strenuous flows. It is also a great pose for beginning a yoga session to open up the back and soothe the adrenals.

Meditation Tips

Like Vata types, Pittas similarly have a tough time meditating. However, unlike Vatas, who may be daydreaming about travels or stressing about situations that haven't even happened, Pittas are planning their schedules, thinking of business ideas, and strategizing their next moves. They are very practical thinkers and sometimes have a hard time understanding what the whole fuss is about meditation. For them, they have to see it to believe it.

At the beginning, they may be completely resistant to meditation. Their left-brain rationality doesn't permit it, and they don't see the benefit of sitting there and doing nothing. In fact, this sounds entirely counterproductive to them. They would much rather use that time doing something that will get them somewhere.

However, once they begin practicing meditation, they fall in love with it. It becomes the missing piece of their lives that finally enables them to become more deliberate and effective in their every move. It creates space in their chaotic minds and allows them, just for a few moments, to become totally still. This presence becomes addictive for them.

Because Pittas are very hard-working, they often become meditation masters. They practice many forms of meditation, from 10-day silent retreats, called Vipassana, to Osho Dynamic Meditation, which involves screaming, dancing, and jumping.

Pittas often can be extremists; they may go from not believing in something to becoming addicted to it. It is especially important for Pittas to cultivate balance in their minds. They don't need to trek to the Himalayas, shave their heads, and walk on fire to gain spiritual wisdom. All they have to do is become more present in their day-to-day actions. That means not becoming angry when they're stuck in traffic, not becoming impatient when someone is taking a long time to learn something, or not snapping when someone asks them the same question for the thousandth time. These are all forms of meditation in practice.

It might sound easy to abandon life and become a meditation master on top of a mountain where no one can bother you. What's difficult is living in that presence today, when you're stuck in traffic, missed your flight, or dealing with a broken-down car. This is when you need true meditation most.

I want to walk you through a guided meditation practice for releasing emotions. The visualization method is especially great for Pittas who need something more realistic to envision in their meditation and can't really grasp things like a white light entering your third eye or Earth's energy coming through your body.

Before you begin, find a comfortable place to sit. I suggest reading the whole meditation through once before practicing it with your eyes closed, at your own pace. Allow any emotions to arise without judgment. It's safe to feel all the feelings, and the only way to get over something is to get through it.

Close your eyes, and take a few breaths. Breathe deeply into your heart center, filling your chest with air. Slowly exhale. Again deeply inhale, making your inhale longer and slower. Hold your breath in, and slowly exhale, making your exhale as long as your inhale. Pause and repeat, lengthening your inhale and exhale with every breath. Continue until you feel like you are in a complete state of peace.

Envision yourself walking on a beach, the cool breeze on your skin, the sand between your toes. You stare out into the deep blue water and see the vastness of the ocean. You surrender to its greatness, feeling how small you are compared to its breadth.

Look down at your feet and notice the waves splashing before you, coming and receding with no end. Some waves are stronger and others are more subtle, but they always continue in the same pattern.

Now imagine your emotions are those waves, ebbing and flowing like an ocean tide. Sometimes it's anger; at other times it's joy. Instead of identifying with a single emotion and letting it stay, watch it go by. Don't attach to a single feeling, just watch them, just witness their transition.

Sadness can turn into laughter. Fear can turn into love. You are not your emotions but rather the space-holders for them. Different tides will come, but you are as vast as the ocean and can remain still, even when the tides change.

Kapha Practices

Kaphas are creatures of habit. If you are a Kapha, perhaps your daily routine has been the same your entire life. You stick to things you believe work. You'd rather maintain certainty than risk trying something new.

Kaphas often have the same friends and live in the same place as they did in their childhood years. For them, the toughest thing is letting go. Kaphas tend to hold on to the past, which can make them accumulate material possessions, too. Their life's practice is detachment, stimulation, and forgiveness.

Kaphas benefit from shaking out their routines and stepping out of their comfort zones. Whereas Vatas are scattered and Pittas are overly structured, Kaphas sometimes can be lazy. They often don't use their time effectively, preventing them from achieving what they want. They'll look back on a weekend they had so many plans for and yet got almost nothing accomplished. Kaphas must work on stimulating, letting go, and practicing every day so they can become all they were meant to be.

Here's an example of a great daily routine for Kapha:

> Wake up before the sun rises to get your day started bright and early.
>
> Practice your morning routine: eliminate, brush teeth, scrape tongue, wash face, oil pull with sesame oil.
>
> Drink a hot cup of warming tea, such as ginger, cinnamon, and cayenne, and meditate.
>
> Get some exercise. Practice sun salutations briskly to activate all channels of your body.
>
> Wait until you're genuinely hungry to eat breakfast. Eat something warm and light, like oatmeal with almond milk and cinnamon. Avoid dairy and pastries.
>
> Get your hardest task of the day done in the morning.
>
> Wait until you're hungry again to eat lunch.
>
> Avoid snacking throughout the day, and wait 4 to 6 hours for your next meal.
>
> Take a brisk walk in nature.
>
> Eat an early, light, easy-to-digest dinner, like vegetable soup.
>
> Enjoy a nightly warm tonic, oil your body with sesame oil, and turn off all technology.
>
> Get to sleep soundly by 10 P.M.

Move Your Body

Kaphas' true medicine is to move their bodies. Kaphas can become stuck, physically and mentally, which causes them to store weight and emotional pain. The antidote for their heaviness is movement.

The best time for Kaphas to move is first thing in morning because that sets them up for the rest of the day. They'll be much more active and achieve much more after they've gotten their sweat session in bright and early. Their metabolisms will be running faster for the rest of the day, too. However, this may be the last time Kaphas want to exercise. Kaphas like to sleep in and are often groggy for the first hour of the day. To shake out of that rut, it's crucial for Kaphas to exercise.

Kaphas require the most vigorous exercise of all the Doshas. They should practice an activity that brings their body to a light sweat. It can be a Vinyasa or power yoga class, a brisk walk, an aerobics class, or cycling. Whatever gets them up and moving is the right type of exercise. They also should be sure to vary their routines to keep their bodies in a state of shock and continually burning fat.

Try New Things

Kaphas like to stick with what they know, which is why it is especially important for them to try something totally new. This allows Kaphas to come out of their comfort zones and expand as individuals. If you do the same thing, day after day, year after year, you won't grow. It is only through that uncomfortable feeling of putting yourself out there that you learn and develop. Kaphas resist that feeling because it is scary for them. But it's what they need to do for their souls to expand.

> **WISDOM OF THE AGES**
>
> Every week, think of one new thing you can do. It can be trying a new workout, visiting a local park, signing up for a new class, meeting a new friend, or taking a solo trip. Whatever it is, become comfortable with the uncomfortable. Growth does not happen when you feel safe and secure. It takes some pushing to expand, but it's always worth it. A butterfly never looks back and says it wishes it remained a caterpillar.

Practice Forgiveness

Kapha types don't forget. They'll remember that time you forgot to call them on their birthday 5 years ago. They'll never let you know, but it stays with them. Kapha types retain emotions, memories, possessions, and even weight. To release that all, they must practice forgiveness.

It's only through forgiveness that you move on. If you don't let go of the things that have hurt you, you'll always be run by those hurts and bring those wounds into future relationships. Forgiveness cuts the cord and allows those things from the past to remain in the past.

Think of all those who have done you wrong, or maybe who you have done wrong. Think of all that miscommunication, jealousy, greed, or anger that got in the way of other, better things in your life. With your whole heart, forgive those people. You can write out a forgiveness note and mail it, or don't, or you can just say it out loud several times. Whether they ever read or hear it is unimportant. What matters is that energetically you have forgiven them and now you are free to move on.

You will feel lighter in your everyday life because you're no longer holding on to that anger or sadness. Mental strain becomes physical strain and by practicing forgiveness, you can break those bonds to become free and light again. You may notice that your weight slips off, too, after you've truly let go of your past—double win!

Yoga Practices

Kaphas like to take things slow and easy, but their yoga practice should be more dynamic and flowing. Kaphas should open their practices to more active forms of yoga, such as Vinyasa or power yoga. Kaphas have the still and calm part down, but what they need is the strength and vitality. Deep stretches also are great to open tensed muscles and joints, especially the hips.

Chaturanga Push-up: A chaturanga push-up, or *chaturanga dandasana,* is like a normal push-up but instead of having your arms out wide, they're placed on either side of your chest with your elbows tucked in alongside your body.

To practice, get your body into push-up position with your arms on either side of you, facing forward. (If this is too intense, you can have your knees down on the floor.) Slowly lower your body with your elbows tucked in, facing backward. Keep your body in a straight line without collapsing your chest or hips forward. Once you've reached your maximum point, slowly push your body back up with your arms in the same position.

This movement works your hard-to-reach triceps area, which is where Kapha types often deposit fat. Practice this in your sun salutations to rev up your metabolic fire.

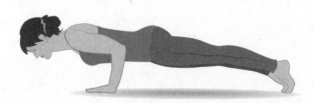

In the chaturanga position, your feet should be approximateily hip width apart. Elbows are bent, but not beyond bringing the shoulders in line horizontally with the elbows. Tighten the thighs, buttocks and abs.

Cobra pose: Cobra pose, also called *bhujangasana*, opens your chest, tones your abdominal walls, and brings suppleness to your spine. In fact, the ancient yoga text Gheranda Samhita says the serpent goddess Kundalini awakens your spine and brings it limberness when you practice cobra pose regularly, hence the name. Cobra pose is the perfect follow-up to chaturanga.

Cobra pose is a heart-opener, meaning it helps open any stored tension in your heart area and allows you to be more loving, receptive, and open. It also strengthens your pancreas and liver, which helps your body remove toxins and shed fat.

This pose can be practiced anytime, just not on a full stomach because it can make you feel a bit nauseated.

To practice, lie on your belly with your head turned to the side. Press your hands into the floor and breathe out. When you breathe in again, slowly lift your upper body by pushing down on your hands. Keep your shoulders down and your elbows close in, as in chaturanga. Keep your head looking straight. Your lower body below your naval should remain on the floor. Press until the point you feel comfortable. There should be no tension in your lower back but a stretch in your upper and middle spine. If it's too much for you, remain on your forearms. Just go to your point of comfort and hold it for about 10 seconds. Slowly lower your body back down and exhale, facing your head in the opposite direction. Repeat two more times.

As you practice cobra pose more, you'll notice your backbend gets deeper and your chest becomes more expansive. You are activating your inner cobra!

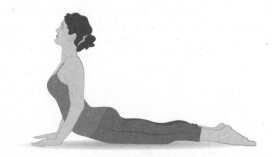

Cobra pose is one of the best poses for increasing spine flexibility, opening the chest and strengthening the shoulders. It also opens the lungs, heals asthma, and stimulates the abdominal organs, enhancing digestion.

Abdominal Twist: The abdominal twist, or *jathara parivartanasana*, helps get things moving, mentally and physically. When you twist your body, you stimulate your digestive system. This helps you digest any rotting food that may have been stuck in your gut. Abdominal twists help wring out toxins, too. They also help strengthen your oblique and core muscles.

There are many ways to practice twists, from lying down to sitting down to being in a lunge. The easiest way involves lying down: lie on your back, and hug your knees into your chest. Slowly bring both knees to the left side of your body. Feel the stretch through the right side of your body, and keep your shoulders on the ground. You should feel an opening in your lower back, side, and shoulder. Allow your body to soften into the stretch, really twisting your internal organs and flushing out any toxins. With each exhale, twist a little deeper. When you're ready, switch your legs over to the right side and repeat.

This is a great stretch to do after a sweaty yoga class when your muscles need a break. It's very expansive, but at the same time, it's healing and supportive, making it a great choice for Kaphas. You also can make this into an oblique exercise by lowering your legs to one side with control, bringing them back up, and lowering them to the other side, repeating back and forth.

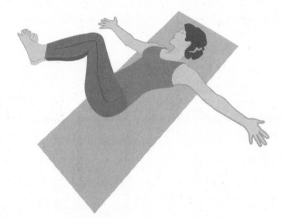

The abdominal twist strengthens digestion by improving the function of the liver, pancreas and small intestine. It also stimulates elimination and the reproductive system.

Meditation Tips

Kapha types are patient and sedentary, but that doesn't mean they're always in a meditative state. In fact, Kaphas are often too stuck in the past to really be present in the moment. It's essential for Kaphas to cultivate a meditation practice so they can become emotionally free.

As a Kapha, you might do well with a walking meditation because it gets your body moving but at the same time keeps you mindful. Before performing a walking meditation, first become aware of your breath. Inhale and exhale until you come to a point of stillness.

Feel your feet on the floor. Feel your legs, your hips, your stomach, your back, your shoulders, your arms, your neck, and your head. Feel all parts of your body and their interconnectivity. Once you have achieved body awareness, slowly take one step while inhaling. Allow that step to be as slow and gradual as possible. After you have shifted weight on your feet, take a second step, exhaling. Continue this process, inhaling and exhaling on each step. Allow your movement to become your meditation.

Practice for 10 minutes a day. This helps you cultivate mind-body awareness, which helps you in your exercise routine and everyday life.

Pranayama

Kaphas often have respiratory issues and can really benefit from *pranayama,* mindful breathing practices.

To practice, sit in a comfortable position on the ground, preferably with your legs crossed and back straight. Place your right index finger over your left nostril and your right thumb over your right nostril. Do not press down; just place them there. Close your mouth.

Now press down with your index finger, blocking your left nostril. Deeply inhale with your right nostril. Fully expand that breath, letting it enter your entire body. When you feel like you can't breathe anymore, pause for a few moments. Now lift your index finger and press down with your thumb. Exhale from your left nostril slowly and deliberately. Allow all the air you inhaled to release from your nostril, and fully exhale any stale air in your lungs. Pause and repeat again.

With this practice, you are cleansing your lungs, increasing cognitive function, decreasing stress, and improving mood—all with just mindful, controlled breathing. Practice every morning and night for at least 5 minutes to reap the benefits.

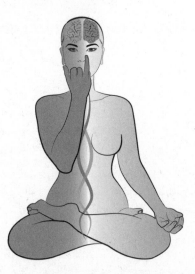

As you practice pranayama, you are circulating energy between the masculine and feminine sides of your brain and body.

WISDOM OF THE AGES

Throughout the day, you switch breathing predominately out of one nostril and then the other. Your body balances your energies by switching your dominant nostril every 90 to 150 minutes. The left nostril is more relaxed and calm, activating the *Ida* nerve ending. It is associated with feminine, yin, changeable, cool, moon energy. The right nostril is more active and alert, activating the *Pingala* nerve ending. It is associated with masculine, yang, hot, sun energy. Notice how your breath switches throughout the day, and observe how you feel. To channel a certain energy, block the other nostril and breathe out of that side for 5 minutes.

The Least You Need to Know

- Each Dosha has particular lifestyle, yoga, and meditation practices beneficial to maintain balance.

- Vatas must work on establishing routine, slowing down, and building their digestive fire. The best yoga practices for Vatas are strengthening, and the key meditations are imaginative and clearing.

- Pittas should focus on chilling out, practicing mindfulness, and staying cool. The optimal yoga practices for Pittas are relaxing and opening, and the best meditations are realistic and visual.

- Kaphas need to move their bodies, try new things, and practice forgiveness to gain balance. The best yoga practices for Kaphas are dynamic and moving, and the ideal meditations are cleansing and focused in the present.

Establishing an Everyday Routine

In Part 3, I teach you how to set up a daily schedule, including a morning and nighttime routine, that gives you optimal energy, digestion, creativity, sleep, and mind-body balance. I also discuss the Ayurvedic practices of self-care, including oil pulling, tongue scraping, and dry brushing. Get ready for some serious self-love!

CHAPTER 9

The Times According to Ayurveda

Time is something we are given every day but never seem to have enough of. We can use our time in countless ways, but not all are conducive to a healthier mind, body, and spirit.

In this chapter, I discuss how you can use Ayurvedic wisdom to set up your daily schedule so you can eat, sleep, digest, work, exercise, and create at your optimal potential, just by following your natural Doshic rhythms.

In This Chapter

- The Ayurvedic times of the day
- Scheduling your day to make the most of the Dosha times
- The best times to eat, sleep, work, dream, and more
- Tips to enhance your life by timing with the Doshas

Categorizing Time

If you had to make a list of the times of the day, what categories would you choose? For most people, it's (quickly eat your) breakfast time, (scarf down your) lunch time, (gorge on) dinner time, and (fall asleep in front of a screen) sleep time, with work sprinkled among the other times.

As a society, you aren't raised to plan our day according to the energy of that particular time. In Spain *siestas,* or nap times, are common to allow Spaniards time to rest after lunch, but here, you work throughout the day, commonly with only a 30-minute lunch break. Dinner is often your biggest meal because it's the only meal you get to eat at home. Few people pack their lunches, and if they do, it's normally a cold sandwich or salad, which is against the Ayurvedic rules of nutrition because cold foods put out digestive fire agni.

You were never taught to schedule your creative tasks in the afternoon, your organized tasks in the morning, and your calming tasks at dusk, as Ayurveda recommends. You just do whatever comes your way without considering how time's energy might affect you. You see each hour as separate from the entire circadian rhythm. You ignore the lunar and solar cycles, which deeply affect your entire beings.

Just like animals come out in the early morning and go to sleep as soon as the sun sets, you, too, are deeply connected with nature. However, your modern way of life has disconnected you, causing you to work and be awake around the clock, leading to imbalances. Ayurveda offers a solution, connecting you daily rhythm with nature's.

Why Follow an Ayurvedic Schedule?

Following an Ayurvedic schedule makes you more effective at all your tasks because you are working with, not against, your own nature. Ayurveda has found that in order for you to function at your optimal potential, you must schedule your days with the solar and lunar cycles. That means rising when the sun rises, building your energy as the sun increases in the sky, eating your biggest meal when the sun is at its peak, and descending your energy with the sun afterward.

Let's look at how you can schedule your day according to the Doshas for optimal health, productivity, and balance.

How the Dosha Times Work

You divide your day into 24 single hours, but Ayurveda splits the day into six 4-hour periods. Each period is related to a certain Dosha and repeats twice throughout the day:

Dosha Times

Kapha times: 6 A.M.- to 10 A.M. and 6 P.M.- to 10 P.M. are associated with Kapha time.

Pitta times: 10 A.M.- to 2 P.M. and 10 P.M.- to 2 A.M. are related to Pitta time.

Vata times: 2 A.M.- to 6 A.M. and 2 P.M.- to 6 P.M. are connected with Vata time.

The rising and falling of the sun is connected to Kapha. Kapha is a grounding earth energy, and as the earth prepares for the day and settles down for night, you are in Kapha time.

The peak of the day and peak of the night are related to Pitta. Pitta is a strong, sharp energy, and the heat of the day and darkness of the night are related to this powerful Dosha.

The transition between night and day and between dusk and dawn is related to Vata. Vata is an ethereal, dreamlike Dosha, and your most active daydreams and nightdreams are both in the Vata times of day.

> **WISDOM OF THE AGES**
>
> The beginning and end of the day, 6-10 A.M. and 6-10 P.M., are associated with Kapha.
>
> The peaks of the day and night, 10 A.M.-2 P.M. and 10 P.M.-2 A.M., are associated with Pitta.
>
> The late hours of the day and night, 2 P.M.-6 P.M. and 2 A.M.-6 A.M., are associated with Vata.

The activities you perform within these hours should be related to the Dosha of that time. As the sun rises and sets during Kapha time, you should focus on settling your body and avoiding all strenuous activity. When the sun is highest in the sky in the first Pitta time, you should do most of your work; in the prime of the night, you should get your highest-quality sleep. In the afternoon and early hours of the morning, you should use your natural creativity for good.

Operating with the Doshas makes you more efficient at everything you do because you finally are working with your own nature.

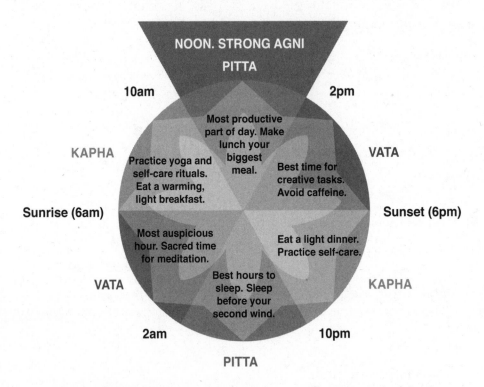

By aligning your days with the natural Doshic rhythms, you will experience optimal digestion, productivity, rest and spiritual awareness.

Kapha Time (6 A.M. to 10 A.M.)

You start the day in the Kapha period. Kapha is earth energy, the time when the sun rises and begins its cycle. You similarly should feel grounded, peaceful, and sometimes lethargic in the morning due to the increase of Kapha energy.

If you wake in the morning feeling groggy and exhausted, this is due to an increase of Kapha. Kapha Prakritis are more likely to feel heavy and tired in the morning because their Kapha especially falls out of balance then, but everyone is susceptible to it. In the winter, when the mornings are gray, you are more likely to experience a Kapha imbalance, which is why you don't feel like getting out of bed in the dark winter months. However, according to Ayurveda, how you start the day is how you'll feel for the rest of it.

It's crucial to nourish, awaken, and activate your body during Kapha time so you can have an energized yet peaceful rest of the day. Let's look at some suggestions on ways to balance your energy during Kapha morning time.

Rise Right Before the Sun

Have you ever been up very early in the morning and noticed that the birds tend to chirp right before the sun rises? That's because they're tuned in with Earth's energy. The best time for humans to wake up is right before the sun rises, too. Ayurveda recommends that to start the day in tranquility, you should watch the sun rise in meditation before the stress of the day begins.

Historically, people woke up with the sun for a number of reasons. They didn't have curtains, so when the sun was up, so were they. And most people were farmers so they had to start their days before the sun rose too high in the sky and it would be too hot to work outside. Or they slept not far after it became dark. They didn't have lights, so when the sun set, their candles could only last them so long until it was time to retire. Humans have functioned this way for thousands of years, and your bodies have adapted to this rhythm. In fact, all mammals follow the same cycle. Warm-blooded creatures were designed to rise and rest with the rhythm of the sun because it's the most effective for your energy levels. But with black-out curtains, eye masks, smartphones, bars, and night shifts today, many people sleep in far past the rising hour of the sun and then rest hours after the sun goes down. This throws them off rhythm for the entire day.

WISDOM OF THE AGES

Have you ever slept in very late and felt tired for the rest of the day, even though you got more than enough sleep? That's because your Kapha energy became imbalanced. When you oversleep, your Kapha rises and you feel heavier and more lethargic. For this reason, Ayurveda recommends rising right before the sun to ensure you aren't sleeping during Kapha time to further increase the energy. Sleeping between 6 A.M. and 10 A.M. makes you more tired for the rest of the day.

Get to sleep early so you can wake up early naturally, not force yourself. If you are not getting to sleep until past midnight, it won't be a good idea to become sleep-deprived just so you can wake up before the sun. Ideally, you should be asleep by 10 P.M. so you can wake up by 6 A.M. feeling refreshed, not exhausted.

Move Your Body

After waking up and meditating with the sunrise, the next thing you should do is yoga or another form of light exercise. When you sleep overnight, you don't move your body much for hours at a time. This makes your muscles stiff, causing tightness and aching when you get up. It's key that you awaken, open, and activate your physical body in the morning so you have an awakened, open, and activated mind for the rest of the day. Some sun salutations, other yoga poses, or even jumping jacks should do the trick.

Kapha time is the best time of day to exercise because it takes you out of your heavy Kapha slump. It revs up your metabolism and digestive fire for the rest of the day. If you are not a morning person and waking up and exercising feels like torture, you especially are in need because that is a sign your Kapha is already out of balance. Ayurveda is all about equilibrium, and wherever there is heaviness, you must counterbalance it with lightness and mobility.

> **WISDOM OF THE AGES**
>
> An activated body is an activated mind. Exercising in the morning before breakfast is the best time because it gives you more energy, alertness, metabolic function, and digestive power for the rest of the day.

Eat a Light Breakfast

What do you eat first thing in the morning? Eggs, pancakes, bacon, or pastries? That's the exact opposite of what you need. Your digestion is like a fire that needs to be kindled lightly in the morning because it hasn't been fed all night. Eating a heavy breakfast is like pouring bricks on that fire and putting it out.

Ayurveda recommends you consume a light, easy-to-digest breakfast to start your day on the right foot. If you consume too much in the morning, your body has to expend extra energy just to digest the food, leaving you with less energy for the rest of the day. You'll feel groggy, heavy, and lethargic, and you'll crave more food just to stay awake.

It's best to consume a warming breakfast that's catered to your unique Doshic constitution. An ideal breakfast would be cooked grains (the type depends on your Dosha) with your choice of milk, cinnamon, and seeds. Stewed apples, lentil soup, or mashed sweet potatoes with cinnamon and cardamom are other great breakfast options.

Stay away from croissants, muffins, and any other baked goods, which are too heavy for your body to digest in the early morning hours. Similarly, granola bars, smoothies, and yogurt are marketed as healthy options but will put out your digestive fire because they're cold. Oatmeal, buckwheat, amaranth, millet, or quinoa porridge are much better options.

AYURVEDIC ALERT

Ayurveda does not recommend coffee as part of your daily morning routine with the exception of Kaphas. Starting your day with a cup of coffee is like throwing gas on your digestive fire, which is especially disruptive for Pitta types. Coffee is extremely acidic, overstimulates your mind and body, causes hyperacidity, and leads to heartburn and even ulcers, especially on an empty stomach. Coffee is also not recommended for Vatas because it dehydrates your body, causing dull skin and premature wrinkles. It may also cause anxiety or insomnia, another issue Vatas suffer from. Only Kaphas can have a small amount of coffee to get them going in the morning, though it shouldn't be a source of dependence.

Pitta Time (10 A.M. to 2 P.M.)

You awaken in Kapha with your chai lattes and then the fire kicks in—it's Pitta time. As the sun rises in the sky, your energy builds. You are able to accomplish the most difficult tasks of the day by harnessing this solar energy. By noon, the sun is highest in the sky and your digestive fire is similarly most active, making it the best time to digest meals.

Pitta time is a period of mental and digestive power, and you should make the most of this by scheduling your hardest tasks and biggest meal now.

At the same time, you have to be careful not to burn yourself out when your energy is high so you can maintain enough for the rest of your day.

Stay Present

It's easy to become overwhelmed with the tasks of the day first thing when you enter the office. Maybe you immediately throw yourself into a task before really scheduling your day. Pitta is an organized energy and works best when you have a plan.

Instead of stressing out about the million things you have to get done in a day, maintain the presence you cultivated in the morning. As the day goes by and you're ticking tasks off your to-do list, you'll be able to get more done by focusing on one task at a time and staying present with that job. When the day gets too hard, just come back to your breath. Don't just start your day in meditation; maintain your day in meditation.

Tackle Your Hardest Task

When your Pitta energy is up and you're in the flow of things, it's the best time to get your hardest tasks out of the way. If you have any organizational or logistical work to do, Pitta is the perfect time for it.

During the Pitta period, you take on the fiery Dosha's qualities, making you more methodical, structured, and logical. Use that in your favor by accomplishing those tasks that require you to use more of your analytical left brain. Pitta time is not great for creative work because your mind hasn't been awake long enough to get into the creative space and is ruled by fire still. Instead, get things done now. Achieve your toughest tasks in this fiery block so you don't have to worry about them for the rest of the day.

Make Lunch Your Biggest Meal

Many of you cram in a quick wrap or salad between meetings during your short lunch break or even eat at your desks while still working. This is a big no-no in Ayurveda.

Rather than eating whatever you can find to hold you over until dinner, you should make lunch the main meal of your day. I know this is difficult because you're probably not home during lunch, but just packing a meal from home to reheat at the office makes a huge difference in your day and your digestion.

Lunch is prime time for eating because your digestive fire is the most active when the sun is highest in the sky. This makes your body most efficient at breaking down food, absorbing nutrients, and eliminating waste.

> **WISDOM OF THE AGES**
>
> Test it out for yourself. One day, make lunch your biggest meal and another day, make dinner your large meal. Notice how much more energy you have, and how much better you sleep, on the days you had a big lunch and small dinner versus the other way around.

Ayurveda recommends eating grains every day, and the best time to do that is midday, when your body is active and can burn off the carbs as energy rather than store them as fat. Additionally, if you eat meat, which is very heavy and difficult to digest, give your body at least 6 hours to digest it. Sleeping on a full stomach is a huge digestive no-no and leads to weight gain, toxicity, bad bacteria overgrowth, and a host of other imbalances.

Use the power of the sun and your digestive fire in your favor, and make lunch the main event of your day. You won't be very hungry for dinner, and a simple soup will suffice, lulling you (and your smaller waistline) right to sleep.

Vata Time (2 P.M. to 6 P.M.)

Between 2 P.M. and 6 P.M., we enter visionary Vata time. This is a time of creativity, lightness, and movement. Your nervous system is the most active then, and it's the best time of day to get your creative tasks done to harness this airy energy.

At the same time, it's often when you feel exhausted and reach for an afternoon pick-me-up cup of coffee or sweet snack. For that reason, you must maintain your energy without reaching for an external source that will actually leave you feeling more depleted in the long run.

Tap into Your Creativity

Vata makes you highly innovative, so this is the best time to focus on your creative tasks. The afternoon Vata period is a great opportunity for writing, producing, designing, and planning future endeavors. By the afternoon, you have boosted your mental energy from building Kapha and stimulating Pitta periods, and now you're ready to think outside the box in imaginative Vata time.

This is also when you may start daydreaming, especially if you're at a job you do not enjoy. It is essential that you work on a project you enjoy that's fulfilling your *dharma*, or life path, so you utilize your daydreams for a positive purpose. Daydreaming can allow you to come up with great insights when you are aligned with your path.

Stay Grounded

Blood sugar levels can crash in the afternoon, and sometimes you might think you need an extra cup of caffeine to stay alert. This is actually the worst thing you can do from an Ayurvedic perspective. When Vata energy is up, it's important you ground down. Coffee will make you more anxious, jittery, and in-your-head, which is the opposite of what you need at this time.

> **WISDOM OF THE AGES**
>
> Instead of taking a walk to the local coffee shop during your lunch break, walk to a nearby park. Slip off your shoes, and connect your feet to the earth in a process called *earthing* or *grounding*. Earth has a slightly negative charge, so when you walk barefoot on the soil, the earth's electrons flow through your body, transmitting its healing power. Earth's ions serve as natural antioxidants, helping your immune system, circulation, and other physiological processes function. Avoid caffeinated beverages, and opt for earthy herbal teas like ginger, dandelion, or rooibos instead. Practice grounding yoga poses like yogi squats (*malasana*) and meditation practices like connecting to your root chakra to ground down your energy (more on chakras in Chapter 21).

Snack Smart, Not Sweet

The afternoon is when you might reach for a something sweet to keep your energy levels up. If you didn't consume a filling lunch, you might indulge in a sugar-laden vending-machine granola bar or cookie (which both often have just about the same amount of sugar) just to stay alert.

Consuming cold and raw foods like salads makes you more likely to crave something sweet and grounding afterward because your body naturally wants to contrast the cool and dry energy. That's why you should add something naturally sweet, like grains, squash, or sweet potatoes to your meals to prevent sugar cravings.

Rather than brownies and banana bread, snack on something high in protein and low in sugar. Smart options include nuts, seeds, soup, avocados, roasted vegetables, and hummus. Keep a healthy snack handy so you don't reach for whatever is available in the closest vending machine when hunger hits. Ayurveda does not recommend snacking, so try to eat substantial meals that hold you over until the next one.

> **WISDOM OF THE AGES**
>
> Only snack if you are truly hungry. Ayurveda does not encourage snacking because it interferes with your body's detoxification process. It's only between the digestion of meals that your body can detoxify, and it takes about 4 hours. If you are continually eating during the day without waiting at least 4 hours between meals, you don't give your body time to detox. Make your lunch filling so you don't need a snack in the afternoon. If you do need something to tide you over, wait at least 4 hours after your last meal. Vatas need snacks the most, followed by Pittas, and lastly Kaphas, who ideally won't snack at all.

Kapha Time (6 p.m. to 10 p.m.)

The second Kapha time of day is when the sun sets and you prepare your body for sleep. It is a peaceful, relaxing span with sunsets and a long-awaited homecoming. This Kapha period is when you should eat dinner, settle your body, practice self-care, and head to bed. By making use of this peaceful energy, you'll have a long, sound night of restorative sleep.

Settle Down

After a tough day at work, you need some practices to help you settle down into the night. Many people take the stress of their days home with them, where it does not belong. You must actively practice mindfulness so you leave the stress of the office at the office. In the evening, you come home not only to your physical home but also back into yourself.

Kapha evenings are best spent in self-care. Whether it is taking a bath, stretching your body, meditating, spending time with your family, cooking dinner, or taking a walk, find a way of calming your mind and body to prepare for rest. The evening is also a great time to make facial masks and massage your body with oil in a practice called *abhyanga* (more on self-oil massage in Chapter 11).

WISDOM OF THE AGES

The brain and body prepare to sleep hours before your actual bedtime. Soothe the body with self-care practices and relax your mind with a 1 or 2 hour technology detox where all screens are put away.

Anything can be performed in a meditative state, from chopping vegetables to helping your kids with homework. All it takes is absolute presence. Listening to disturbing news stories or sitting in front of the television is neither self-care nor mindful. Avoid activities that are overly stimulating or negative, and instead bring the focus back to yourself and your surroundings. If you do not make a purposeful point to practice presence and take care of your body, you'll lose sight of who you truly are.

Eat a Light Dinner

Most people make dinner their biggest meal of the day, and understandably so—it may be the only meal they get to eat at home. However, this is no excuse to gorge on dinner that will end up leaving you feeling stuffed until the next day.

Ayurveda recommends consuming a light, easily digestible supper such as a roasted vegetable soup, spiced lentils, or grains so your body can quickly digest the meal before you go to sleep. If you eat something overly heavy, such as fried foods, meat, pasta, cheese, or bread, you don't give your body enough time to break down the meal, and instead, it's stuck in your gastrointestinal tract overnight.

AYURVEDIC ALERT

When you eat a heavy dinner, your body does not have time to digest the meal before you go to sleep, meaning the food sits in your gastrointestinal tract and putrefies. This fermentation often leaks into your blood stream and spreads toxicity throughout your entire body. Toxicity symptoms look different for each Dosha, but they can be anything from bloating and gas to acne and anxiety, depending on your Doshic constitution. Avoid these symptoms by having a light dinner.

During Kapha time, your digestive fire is not as strong because your body is preparing for sleep. Therefore, the foods you eat aren't broken down in time, and they're more likely to be stored as fat. This also can cause excess bad bacteria in your stomach, leading to candida, small intestinal bacterial overgrowth (SIBO), and other related digestive disorders. Keep dinner light and simple so you can wake up feeling refreshed, not food-hungover.

Walk After Your Meal

Ayurveda recommends taking a short walk for about 15 minutes after your meal to aid your digestion and help regulate your elimination. Too often you might sit down after a big meal and not really move again until the next day. Simply walking around your house, up and down your hallway, or ideally around your block is all you need. It does not have to be strenuous. Ask a family member along for company.

Getting into the habit of walking after your meal enhances longevity, improves digestion, and increases your metabolism. If you've eaten so much you can't get off the couch, then chances are you've overeaten. After a well-digested meal you should feel light and energized, not heavy and lethargic.

Pitta Time (10 P.M. to 2 A.M.)

If you're a night owl like me, you may have noticed you get a second burst of energy around 10 P.M. This is when you enter Pitta time. Pitta is a time of activity (and appetite), which is why if you aren't in bed before 10, you'll suddenly get another rush of alertness and perhaps appetite as well. Parents know to get their kids in bed before this second wind kicks in because otherwise the little ones will be up all night.

> **WISDOM OF THE AGES**
>
> Ever noticed that you get a second wind around 10 P.M.? That's because it's Pitta time. Get in bed before 10 P.M. to avoid a midnight frenzy.

Many young adults use this Pitta surge of energy to engage in social activities or hit the library and study. Bars and nightclubs operate specifically at this time, opening at 10 P.M. and shutting down at 2 A.M. Coincidence? I think not. All people are affected by the Doshic time shifts, even if they have no idea what they are.

If you don't plan on hitting the club or library and have somewhere to be in the morning, avoid this second wind by turning off your lights by 10 P.M. This might seem like an impossible task, but it actually can be easy if you've used the Kapha period beforehand to wind down your body.

Many of us get frustrated when we can't fall asleep. Spending time on your computer and actively engaging in work at night fires up your brain. The moment you turn off your laptop, you expect your mind to power down, too, but it doesn't work that way. Your body requires gradual shifts to prepare for the next task. The following suggestions help you make the most of your Pitta time through deeply relaxing sleep.

Turn Off Electronics

How attached are you to your electronics? Do you wake up and immediately grab them to reconnect to the world? Do you go to sleep cuddled up with your smartphone? If so, you're not alone. However, by doing so, you are exposing yourself to blue light, the backlight color of these screens. According to *Scientific American,* the light from our devices is "short-wavelength-enriched," meaning it has a higher concentration of blue light than natural light. This blue-tinted light shifts your body's natural clock and can reduce your natural levels of melatonin, the sleep-inducing hormone.

Your body is naturally affected by the light around you. When the sun is up, your energy is up and your melatonin levels are down. As the sun goes down, your energy depletes and your melatonin levels rise to prepare you for bed. However, if you are constantly staring into a screen, you are exposing yourself to light at all times. Your body doesn't know when it's time to sleep, and it doesn't produce the right hormones. Effectively, you scramble your body's circadian rhythm, and you're left feeling wired and awake in the middle of the night.

WISDOM OF THE AGES

Schedule a technology-free period for at least 1 hour before bed. Instead of reading articles on your screen, read them in a book, magazine, or newspaper. If you absolutely must be on an electronic device, switch it to night mode, which has an orange-tinted background instead of blue. Dim the lights, and light some relaxing candles so you can help nudge your body toward sleep. You have to give your body clues that it's time to rest because sleep doesn't come with a push of a button. It's an interrelated process that comes after a full cycle of the Dosha times.

Turn Off Your Mind

Unfortunately, your brain doesn't come with an off switch so you must have some sort of pre-sleep meditation practice to prepare yourself for a night of rest. Head to bed, light some candles, turn on your essential oil diffuser, read a book—whatever you need to do to put your body in a relaxed state so it can drift off to sleep. Even if you aren't tired, head to bed and perform your nightly ritual so you can train yourself to go to sleep before you get your second wind.

Be sure you're tucked in bed before your fire reignites at 10 P.M. and you start organizing your house or cleaning your closets in your second Pitta rush. I can't count the number of times my clock strikes 10 o'clock and I decide to take on the remainder of the day's tasks I didn't finish instead of going to bed and waking up the next morning to do them during productive Pitta time (10 A.M. to 2 P.M.).

Whatever comes up at night, write it down and forget about it for the night. Tomorrow, you can get to it when the sun is up and on your side. Night is meant for sleeping. There is more than enough time for everything to be done, as long as you stick to your routine.

The Importance of Sleep

All this prepares you for your most important function of the day—sleep. Sleep is the most restorative, healing part of your day. You might stress about diet and exercise but maybe don't think twice about your sleep quality. Sleep is when you restore your muscles, detoxify your body, balance your hormones, relax your mind, and prepare your body and your mind to take on the next day.

However, most people don't get enough sleep. The National Sleep Foundation reports that 60 percent of Americans have sleep problems a few nights a week or more. Not sleeping well can make you feel lethargic the next day and be more likely to overeat due to an increase of ghrelin, the appetite-increasing hormone.

You may have noticed that you're hungrier the day after a sleepless night. That's not just your imagination; you really do get hungrier due to hormonal shifts in your body. A lack of sleep is associated with increased appetite, leading to weight gain. A 2004 study published in *PLOS Medicine* found that short sleep duration is associated with reduced leptin, elevated ghrelin, and increased body mass index. That means that even if you're eating healthy and exercising regularly, if you're not getting enough sleep, you'll still gain weight.

 AYURVEDIC ALERT

If you are trying to lose weight, make sure you're sleeping enough. When you are lacking in sleep, you are more likely to overeat and gain weight.

Lack of sleep is only one part of the equation; quality of sleep is the other, which I explain next. Now, get to bed before your second Pitta wind to ensure you're getting your 8 hours.

Get Quality Sleep Before Midnight

You might think sleep is sleep, but not all sleep is equal. The rest you get from a nap is not as healing as what you get from a full night's sleep. Waking up throughout the night won't give you the same slumber as sleeping soundly for a full 8 hours, either.

The reason is because you go through REM cycles in your sleep. These are stages in your sleep, around 90 to 120 minutes each, that reoccur throughout the night. *REM* stands for "rapid eye movement," and during these sleep cycles, you have sudden eye movements related to your dreams. The longer you've been asleep, the deeper the REM cycle, and the more healing and restorative your sleep.

> **WISDOM OF THE AGES**
>
> According to Ayurveda, the sleep you get before midnight is the most healing of the night. When the sun sets, the earth's atmosphere retains solar energy until around midnight. Your sleep during this residual solar energy is highly nourishing and heal-ing. If you get to sleep right before Pitta time begins at 10 P.M., you can sleep soundly throughout this high-quality resting period before midnight and reap its benefits.

Vata Time (2 A.M. to 6 A.M.)

The final, or really primary, period of the day is Vata time between 2 A.M. and 6 A.M. This is a time of deep dreaming, believed to be when the veils between the universe and Earth are lifted. You can gain deep insights during this auspicious hour, which is why Kundalini yoga meditation practices advocate waking up at 2 A.M. to practice *kriyas,* or chanting.

The early morning is a quiet time when the world is asleep and you can get deeper into your psyche without distraction. You also become in tune with your creative Vata energy during these hours, which is why many artists stay up all night to create or wake very early in the morning to work.

The Veil Between Earth and Universe Is Lifted

The early hours of the morning are especially auspicious because it is believed the veil between the earth and the universe is lifted during this time. This allows for tremendous insights because you are more connected with your higher self. Your mind becomes clearer, and you can tap into your universal brain, which connects you with the spirit and the entire cosmos. For this reason, many meditation practices are done in the early Vata hours to receive the deep insights attained during this time.

Sacred Time for Meditation

The best time of day for a meditation practice is in the early morning before the sun rises. You have yet to begin the tasks of your day and are more centered and in the moment.

Ayurveda recommends rising right before the sun so you can spend some time in silence, observing the stillness of the earth. When the sun rises, you enter Kapha time again, and the cycle repeats.

The Least You Need to Know

- Ayurveda categorizes time into six 4-hour periods, each led by a Dosha that repeats itself in the morning and night.
- The hours between 6 A.M. and 10 A.M. and again between 6 P.M. and 10 P.M. during dusk and dawn are grounding Kapha hours. You'll feel calm and peaceful, preparing to begin and end your day.
- The hours between 10 A.M. and 2 P.M. and again between 10 P.M. and 2 A.M. are high-functioning, achievement-oriented Pitta hours. Tackle your hardest tasks and eat your biggest meal during the midday Pitta hours, and get high-quality sleep during the late-night hours.
- The hours between 2 A.M. and 6 A.M. and again between 2 P.M. and 6 P.M. are creative, auspicious Vata hours when you are more connected with your imaginative and spiritual sides. Take advantage of the afternoon Vata shift for artistic and inventive tasks, and use the early morning period for dreaming and meditation.

CHAPTER 10

Setting Up Your Morning Routine

Every day you rise, you are given a new chance to create your ideal day. In Ayurveda, it is believed that the way you start your day is how you will feel for its duration. If you start your day stressed and rushed, you'll subconsciously feel hurried and agitated for the rest of the day. If you begin your day with inner peace and tranquility, you will take on that mindfulness for the day's duration.

In this chapter, I share ways you can set up your morning routine to maintain that blissed-out feeling all day. With some simple practices, you can cultivate balance, detoxify your body, increase your energy levels, stimulate your metabolism, enhance your digestion, and prevent cravings so you can go through your day with awareness and presence. All it takes is adding 30 minutes to your morning to reap these benefits and have a more productive and centered day.

In This Chapter

- Why you need a morning routine
- Scrape your tongue to detoxify your body
- The what, why, and how of oil pulling
- Starting your day with something hot

The Importance of Your Morning Routine

Your daily routine is called *dinacharya* in Sanskrit. *Din* means "day," and *acharya* means "to follow" or "close to." As mentioned in Chapter 9, you should follow the rhythm of the sun to best support your body's natural functions. The early morning hours are most essential for setting the tone for the rest of the day.

After a long night's rest, you must awaken, open, and activate each channel of your body so you can begin your day on the right foot. If you do not take the time to stimulate your senses and detoxify your body in the morning, you will carry heaviness and toxicity for the rest of the day.

> **DEFINITION**
>
> **Dinacharya** means "to follow or be close to the day." By establishing a routine in line with the natural rhythm of the day, you can accentuate your digestion, sleep, and other functions. Ayurveda believes that your daily routine is of utmost importance. Establishing a healing morning routine cleanses the body of toxins that have accumulated overnight and prepares your mind and body to take on the day.

How Your Mornings Set Your Day

Have you ever woken up to the sound of your alarm, looked at your clock, and realized you'd overslept? You jumped out of bed, hurriedly got dressed, and ran out of the door, maybe grabbing a granola bar for some kind of nourishment for the day.

You may have noticed things just felt off for the rest of that day. You ended up stuck in a traffic jam on your way to work, spilled coffee on your shirt right before an important meeting, and got a task list from your boss that may take you another lifetime to complete. Nothing seemed to be going your way.

You came home from the stressful day and decided to eat something delicious (and naughty) to ease the tension. Before you knew it, you were knee-deep in the peanut butter jar and were binging on things you *know* you weren't supposed to touch. However, you continued eating—anything sweet or salty to get your mind off the stress you were feeling. Only when you finished, you felt even worse than when you began.

This is what emotional eating looks like, caused by only a rushed morning.

Now, have you ever woken up with ample time before your first commitment and given yourself the opportunity to begin the day in mindfulness? Before even opening your eyes, you connected with your dreams and said your gratitude, cultivating peace in your mind. You slowly arose from bed and stretched out your body like a cat waking from a nap. You headed to the bathroom to eliminate, brush your teeth, scrape your tongue, and wash your face without the pressure of the clock. Before looking through your phone and answering emails, you sat yourself down for meditation to silence your mind and give yourself the gift of a few tranquil minutes before the day began. You then headed to the kitchen to make a hot glass of herbal tea and wrote down your intentions for the day.

For the rest of the day, you felt disciplined, peaceful, patient, loving, and grateful. This is all because you took the time to cultivate these emotions in your morning ritual.

If your mornings sound more like the former rather than the latter, have no fear. In this chapter, I explain how you can set up your morning routine so you are better equipped to cope with the day's pressures with ease and graciousness. By practicing this morning routine, you can undergo your day with awareness, without becoming anxious about the future or longing to change the past. You'll digest your food better and no longer need to self-medicate your stress with emotional eating. You'll feel much more in control of your thoughts, and your energy levels will skyrocket. Let me teach you how.

The Benefits of a Morning Routine

Morning routines have countless mental and physical benefits. The benefits of a morning routine include increased energy, enhanced digestion, improved mood, a detoxified body, increased productivity, a more centered mind, enhanced awareness, an ability to focus, less mental fog, and decreased stress levels.

Many successful people, in all industries, credit their success to a morning practice. You can, too. No matter how busy you are, carve out some time in your schedule for a morning practice.

WISDOM OF THE AGES

Try to have the first hour of your day vary as little as possible with a set routine you practice no matter where you are of how busy life gets. The secret of success is found in your morning routine.

What If You Don't Have Time?

Don't say you don't have time to meditate or take care of your body in the morning. By taking the time to center your mind in the morning, you actually create *more* time in the rest of your day because you will be more effective.

You'll be able to jump into your tasks more quickly without first needing to clear away any mental fog. You will have a renewed sense of productivity when, by 8 A.M., you'll have accomplished more than most people do their entire day. You won't walk into work tired and grumpy but rather refreshed and energized because you've taken that time to awaken your senses. You'll be that person smiling at everyone in the office at 9 A.M. when most people are still struggling to open their eyes.

Most importantly, you'll have that much-needed "me time" before emails pile up, responsibilities must be met, children need taking care of, and tasks must be accomplished. The morning is the perfect time to watch the sun rise and really give gratitude for the beauty of the day. You'll take on a sense of joy and appreciation no matter what is asked of you throughout the day because you've carved out that time in the morning for yourself.

What If You're Not a Morning Person?

It's not difficult to become an early riser, even if you've always been a "night owl." All it takes is practice. The number-one thing is to get to sleep earlier. No matter how hard you try, you'll never be a morning person if you're going to sleep late at night. Prioritize your morning versus your night activities. Was it really worth staying up until midnight to watch that TV show? Did you use your time productively before heading to bed? How many hours did you spend on social media the day before?

There can be enough time in the day to do the things you want to do. You just need to cut back on the things that are keeping you from having time for those tasks.

Ask yourself:

- What things am I doing that I could cut back on?

- How much time do I spend on social media or other distractions?

- How many hours do I devote each week to watching TV or movies?

- What can I shorten or get rid of in my nighttime ritual so I can make time for my morning ritual?

When you've pinpointed your time-wasters, choose one that you will shorten by 15 minutes. Then, go to sleep 15 minutes earlier and wake up 15 minutes earlier. The following week, take another 15 minutes away so you can go to sleep and wake up another 15 minutes earlier. Continue doing this each week until you're getting to sleep by 10 P.M. and waking by 6 A.M. By following this gradual process, you can become a morning person easily and without any drastic changes or force. You first must create space to add the things you need. By removing 15 minutes of activities that aren't serving you well, you can add 15 minutes of things that are.

By following this simple 15-minute plan, in a matter of weeks, you'll naturally become a morning person and much more efficient with your time!

Scheduling Your Morning Routine

Everyone's morning routine will look a little different, but here are some general Ayurvedic guidelines to help you establish yours:

Rise before the sun.

Take a few moments to recall your dreams and express your gratitude.

Rise from bed and gently stretch your body.

Go to the bathroom to evacuate.

Splash your face with warm water six times.

Brush your teeth and scrape your tongue.

Swish oil in your mouth while you're getting ready and boiling water for tea.

Spit out the oil, and rinse your mouth with warm water.

Drink your tea and meditate.

Practice yoga.

Eat a warming breakfast.

Keep in mind you do not exactly have to follow this order, but this gives you an overview of what your morning should look like. Mornings are a time to release toxins through evacuation, tongue scraping, and oil pulling, as well as rev up your agni with hot tea, yoga, and a warming breakfast.

You could add other practices to your morning routine such as *nasya* nasal drops, which is applying oil to your nasal passages, as well as abhyanga, or self-oil massage, which I have included in the upcoming nightly ritual chapter.

Tongue Scraping

If you've ever woken up with bad breath in the morning or seen a white coating on your tongue, you already know how the tongue can be a breeding ground for bad bacteria. Yet most of us quickly brush over our tongue with our toothbrush without paying much attention to this area.

Scraping your tongue is just as important as brushing your teeth. According to Ayurveda, all toxins begin in the mouth. When you let tongue bacteria accumulate, the toxicity spreads down your gastrointestinal tract to the rest of your body. This toxicity, ama, is seen as a white, mucous coating. You can see the coating on your tongue, but you can't see what's spreading within your body.

> **WISDOM OF THE AGES**
>
> Your tongue says a lot about you. Just by observing its color, coating, and the location of the coating, you can determine your Doshic imbalance, and have a better idea of what's going on within.

Mouth and Tongue Toxins

Scraping your tongue is just as essential as brushing your teeth. When you sleep overnight, the bacteria, food debris, fungi, dead cells, and toxins on the surface of your tongue builds. This is why you get morning breath.

If you do not scrape off these toxins every morning, your tongue reabsorbs them and they enter your gastrointestinal tract. This toxicity causes a weakened digestive fire, lowered immune system, and decreased ability to assimilate nutrients, which leads to weight gain, acne, illness, bloating, gas, constipation, and other imbalances, depending on your Dosha.

Tongue scraping improves your dental health, prevents gum infections and recessions, increases immunity, enhances saliva production to break down food, enhances your taste buds, improves digestion, and promotes elimination, making it a great way to start your day.

> **WISDOM OF THE AGES**
>
> Recent dental research has agreed with Ayurveda's ancient findings. Clinical trials have shown that approximately 85 percent of all cases of halitosis (chronically bad breath) have their origin in the mouth, and 50 percent of these are caused by tongue residues. Tongue scraping significantly reduces oral bacteria in the crevices of the tongue and was found to be very important for halitosis management. But do you really need a tongue scraper? Doesn't your toothbrush do a good-enough job? In the study, participants were split between using a tongue scraper or toothbrush to clean their tongues. The tongue scraper performed better in reducing the production of volatile sulfur compounds than the toothbrush.

Digestion Begins on the Tongue

Ayurveda states that you begin digesting the moment you taste your food. Your saliva begins breaking down the specific enzymes in your meal and signals to the rest of your body to prepare for food. Your body intuitively knows what enzymes it needs for starches versus proteins. However, when your tongue is coated, your body has no idea what's going on. This disrupts your digestion and prevents it from functioning properly.

According to Ayurvedic expert Dr. Douillard, taste bud activation from tongue scraping also engages the lower intestines to initiate a complete bowel elimination first thing in the morning. This is extremely important for detoxification so you can release stored-up waste in your bowels and get your digestive fires going in the morning.

Scrape More; Eat Less

Studies have shown that tongue scraping lowers the tongue's microbial load, which makes you more sensitive to tastes. In the study, taste sensation improved after 2 weeks of tongue cleaning, especially with a scraper.

The less tongue coating, the more you can taste your food. Tongue scraping helps you become fuller with less amount of food because you taste the flavors more. Oftentimes people overeat simply because they want more flavor from their food. It's not that they're hungry necessarily but just want more sweet, sour, or salty. By scraping your tongue, you become more sensitive to flavors and don't need to overeat just for taste. You become more satisfied with less food, helping you lose weight as well as promote digestion.

> **WISDOM OF THE AGES**
>
> Want to be able to taste your food better? Then scrape your tongue. By removing the toxic coating of your tongue, your tastebuds become more sensitive, allowing you to be more satisfied with less food.

Types of Tongue Scrapers

Now that you're convinced you need a tongue scraper, let me help you find the best one. I recommend purchasing a tongue scraper made out of stainless steel, though it is not traditionally Ayurvedic. The original Ayurvedic text *Charaka Samhita* recommends a tongue scraper made of either copper, gold, silver, tin, or brass. However, a pure gold or silver tongue scraper is expensive and tin and brass aren't very appetizing, making copper the most popular option. Copper also has great antibacterial benefits and has been used on the bottom of ships to keep the water surfaces sanitary for years.

However, I recommend a stainless steel tongue scraper because unlike copper, it is not a heavy-metal. Heavy metals build up in the tissues, causing heavy metal toxicity. Symptoms include fatigue, mental racing, emotional highs and lows, anxiety and reproductive problems. Women are more prone to copper accumulation because estrogen increase copper retention. You can test for heavy metal toxicity through a hair mineral test, though they don't always detect it. I recommend minimizing your exposure to copper to prevent a potential build-up.

AYURVEDIC ALERT

Stainless steel is the safest option when it comes to tongue scraping because it does not expose you to potential heavy metal toxicity and copper overload, which women are most susceptible to. There are many great U-shaped steel tongue scrapers with comfortable handles available on the market.

How to Scrape Your Tongue

It isn't difficult to tongue scrape. In fact, I think it's much easier than flossing (although it in no way replaces it):

1. Hold the scraper with one hand on each end.

2. Look in a mirror, and stick out your tongue. Place the scraper on the back of your tongue, being careful not to gag yourself.

3. Gently scrape the surface of your tongue in a long stroke from back to front. You'll notice ama, the white mucus, accumulate on the scraper.

4. Repeat 10 times. You see that even the pink spots on your tongue have ama stored in the deep crevices.

5. Rinse the scraper with water, and store in a clean place.

Practice every morning before or after brushing your teeth. Ideally, follow it with oil pulling.

Oil Pulling

Oil pulling is the practice of swishing oil in your mouth to remove toxins, sort of like an ancient mouthwash. Oil pulling has a number of benefits, both in your mouth and in the rest of your body.

On the oral side, oil pulling helps cure tooth decay, improves breath, prevents cavities, whitens teeth, removes stains, heals bleeding gums, and strengthens your gums and jaw. On the digestive side, it helps remove oil-soluble toxins from your system, improves digestion, prevents inflammation, and enhances your immune system.

Types of Oil to Use

What type of oil should you use for oil pulling? That depends on your Dosha:

Vatas: Go for sesame oil, which is especially warming and grounding.

Pittas: Use coconut oil, which is cooling and counterbalances Pitta's fieriness.

Kaphas: Choose sesame oil, which revs up your cool digestive fire.

You can change the oil according to the Dosha of the season if you like. Use sesame oil in the colder months and coconut oil in the warmer months.

How to Oil Pull

Oil pulling might seem like a very foreign concept, but it's actually quite simple. Here's how to do it:

1. Place 1 tablespoon oil in your mouth, and swish it around your mouth for as long as possible. Start with just 2 or 3 minutes, and work your way up to 20 minutes, which is what the Ayurvedic texts recommend.

2. Spit out the oil into the trash. Do not swallow the oil because it's full of your toxins, bacteria, and plaque. Do not spit the oil in the sink if you have a septic system because it can clog your drains.

3. Rinse your mouth with warm water or brush your teeth afterward.

There's no need to stand still while you're oil pulling. You can walk around, get dressed, and perform your regular morning tasks while you're swishing the oil in your mouth. Spit it out when you're ready to drink your morning tea.

> **WISDOM OF THE AGES**
>
> Oil pulling is essentially Ayurvedic mouthwash, replacing chemical-filled mouthwash with soothing oil to refresh your breath for the entire day Unlike commercial mouthwashes, oil only removes the bad bacteria while keeping the good, keeping your mouth balanced.

Drink Something Hot

After you've woken up, brushed your teeth, scraped your tongue, and swished oil around your mouth, it's time to drink something nice and steamy. Ayurveda recommends starting your day with a hot drink because it is more hydrating and healing than something cold. Warm beverages like tea or hot water with lemon cleanse your body, dissolve ama from your system, stimulate your digestive fire, and enhance your metabolism.

Hot Is Hydrating

You may have noticed when you are washing dishes that hot water is much more effective at dislodging debris than cold water. This also holds true in your body. Your body more easily absorbs hot water, making it more accessible and hydrating. Your body does not have to exert any extra energy to warm the water, leaving more energy for healing. Drinking hot, boiled water flushes out your lymphatic system; softens hardened tissues; and dilates, cleanses, and hydrates deep tissues. It also heals and repairs your digestive system and flushes the gut-associated lymphoid tissue (GALT), the lymph on the outside of the intestinal wall.

When you sleep overnight, your body becomes dehydrated. Morning is the time it needs hot water the most. Hot water prevents and treats constipation by hydrating your internal organs, especially important for Vata types. It also hydrates chronically dry skin from within, giving you a vibrant glow.

Hot Stimulates the Digestive Fire

Drinking hot water enhances your digestive fire, the internal flame within you related to metabolism, digestion, and assimilation. When you put cold water on this fire, you essentially put out the flames. On the other hand, when you kindle this fire with hot water, it burns much more brightly for the rest of the day. Subsequently, you are better able to digest, break down, and assimilate your meals, allowing your body to make the most of the energy (calories) you consume and store less as fat. Modern science has found similar research. According to a study by *The Journal of Physiology,* cold water has a negative impact on meal digestion.

Ever noticed that restaurants bring you a glass of ice water before a meal? Say no and instead ask for hot water with lemon. Cold water causes the stomach to contract and become too tight to process food effectively. This inhibits the digestive process, making you feel overly full and bloated after eating. The reason this practice even began was because restaurants wanted clients to feel overly full and satisfied after a meal so they'd feel like they got their money's worth, even if their digestive system is overwhelmed. They don't want you to walk out still feeling like you could eat more, but that's exactly what you should want.

Hot water also allows you to slow down your drinking pace. Many of us drink water far too quickly. Drinking excess water while eating dilutes your stomach acid, making it too weak to break down your meal. Instead of chugging down a big glass of water, take slow sips of hot water throughout the day to maintain hydration.

> **WISDOM OF THE AGES**
>
> Hot water increases your core body temperature and enhances your circulation to facilitate detoxification of potentially harmful toxins in your system. With a cleaner system, you're better able to digest foods and make the most of the nutrients you are consuming. An enhanced digestive fire leads to less cravings, fat reduction, decreased bloat, and clear skin, so sip hot water throughout the day for one week and notice how much more hydrated you feel!

Hot Aids Cleansing

Drinking hot water or herbal tea aids cleansing because it softens the food debris in your system and allows your body to flush fat. When you consume ice-cold water, the food it comes in contact with solidifies and hardens, making the intestines contract tightly. This leads to constipation, bloating, and other gastrointestinal pains.

Similarly, the oils you consume from your food solidify in your body when you drink cold water, turning it into mucus, or ama. This mucus lines the intestines, causing toxicity. Frequent sips of hot water throughout the day help extricate these fat cells and cleanse your system.

Overall, drinking a hot beverage helps your body digest, assimilate, and cleanse better for the rest of the day. Instead of reaching for an iced coffee, tea, or frozen smoothie for breakfast, start your day with something hot for its myriad health benefits.

The Least You Need to Know

- The way you start your day is the way you'll feel for the rest of it.
- Tongue scraping is the ancient Ayurvedic practice of scraping the white toxicity off your tongue in the morning and can be conducted with a copper or stainless steel U-shaped tongue scraper.
- Oil pulling is the ancient Ayurvedic method of mouth-washing, consisting of swishing and gargling sesame or coconut oil in your mouth for up to 20 minutes to dislodge toxins.
- Drinking hot water is more hydrating, stimulating for the digestive fire, and cleansing than cold water, especially before meals.

Ayurvedic Nightly Rituals

Ahh, blessed night, when the sun sets and you can prepare your body for a night of deeply healing sleep. In Ayurvedic times, people came home from a long day of working in the field and spent the duration of the day in self-care, scrubbing their skin, oiling their bodies, and boiling healing elixirs. Then something happened in the past few hundred years that slightly changed things. Now, for many people, nights are filled with long commutes, heart-wrenching news stories, and binge watching Netflix. How much things can change in a few centuries!

But wait! You can go back and reintegrate these healing therapies in your life. It's really quite simple, and all it takes is a little awareness. In this chapter, I teach you how to exfoliate, oil, and cleanse your body with easy practices that will make you feel like you're at an Ayurvedic spa in your very own home. You'll drift off to sleep feeling rejuvenated and relaxed.

In This Chapter

- Setting the mood—and scent—for sleep
- How dry brushing can change your life, and skin, forever
- Soothing your mind and relaxing your muscles with oil
- Cleansing your nostrils (yes, your nostrils!)

Slowing Down for Sleep

The moment you get home from work, you should begin preparing your body for rest. Sleep doesn't come the moment you turn off the lights but rather takes hours of what I like to call "sleep foreplay."

Restful sleep doesn't come easy. You must set the mood in order for your body to be whisked away into la-la land. Think of it as your own personal sleep seduction. In the following sections, I share my favorite Ayurvedic tips to create the atmosphere for a restful night.

Technology Detox

There's nothing less sexy than someone on their phone, totally ignoring you. The same rule applies for sleep. If you are glued to your screen, the subtle layers of your mind won't get the hint that it's time to take off to dream world. Instead, you'll awaken your fight-or-flight signals that say it's time to go, produce, and perform. The last thing your brain will want to do is sleep.

I recommend scheduling a technology detox for at least 1 hour before it's time for bed. When you are exposed to the blue light that emanates from a screen, your melatonin levels decrease, preventing you from falling asleep. Instead of cuddling up with your smartphone, choose a book instead, which doesn't have the same artificial lighting as a screen.

Set the Scent

Turn off the lights, light some candles, and turn on your essential oil diffuser. Sleep doesn't come easy, and you have to work to create the right atmosphere for it to come.

I recommend purchasing an essential oil diffuser and adding a few drops of lavender, chamomile, rose, frankincense, or neroli to soothe your nervous system and prepare your body and mind for sleep. We are so deeply affected by our senses, and practicing aromatherapy has been found to ease the mind, reduce anxiety, eliminate stress, and balance hormones, taking us out of the fight-or-flight response of the day.

Additionally, I suggest you avoid all artificially scented candles, such as the delicious apple pie or pumpkin spice candles available at the mall. According to a South Carolina State University study, the long-term use of paraffin candles may cause health hazards, including cancer, common allergies, and asthma. The candles contain alkanes, alkenes, and toluene, which are proven to have harmful effects on humans. Additionally, scented candles produce more soot than unscented candles, which creates indoor air pollution.

Instead of artificially fragranced paraffin candles, choose all-natural soy candles fragranced with essential oils. By-products of natural soy plants, soy candles generally are not harmful to people. Many homemade essential oil-scented soy candles are available online and in natural markets.

The Benefits of Pink Himalayan Sea Salt

I also recommend purchasing pink Himalayan sea salt candleholders and lights. Sea salt is a natural negative ion generator and has been proven to increase the flow of oxygen to the brain, resulting in higher alertness, decreased drowsiness, and more mental energy, according to Pierce Howard, PhD, author of *The Owner's Manual for the Brain*. He states, "They also may protect against germs in the air, resulting in decreased irritation due to inhaling various particles that make you sneeze, cough, or have a throat irritation." If you've ever noticed how grounded and pure you feel when you're on the beach or by a waterfall, it's because of the negative ions in the air from the water.

> **WISDOM OF THE AGES**
>
> Pink Himalayan sea salt lights make great night-lights because they provide a warm, pink-hued glow, similar to a campfire, easing you to sleep. Even better, they don't have the harsh blue light that interferes with your melatonin levels and prevents you from falling asleep. They improve air quality, soothe allergies, boost mood, and offer light therapy, making them a great choice for those with seasonal affective disorder or anyone with a high-stress lifestyle. Himalayan salt inhalers are even used to treat asthma because the salt purifies the air, removing pollutants and allergens.

No matter what, completely avoid all air fresheners, including plug-ins, gels, and aerosols. These are highly toxic and have been linked to cancer and other diseases.

Nature provides us with so many wonderful smells available in essential oils, and it's best to inhale them naturally, through essential oil diffusers and soy candles with pink Himalayan salt holders.

Dry Brushing

After you've detoxed from technology and introduced a soothing scent, it's time to *dry brush* your body. In this ancient Ayurvedic practice, scrape the dead skin cells off the top layer of your skin by brushing your skin with a dry brush before showering. Dry brushing promotes detoxification and stimulates your lymphatic system.

> **DEFINITION**
>
> **Dry brushing** is the Ayurvedic practice of gently scraping the body with a dry loofa brush to remove toxins and dead skin cells and stimulate the lymphatic system.

Why Dry Brush?

Your skin is your largest organ, and one third of your body's toxins are excreted through your skin. If your skin is covered with dead follicles, it cannot breathe and detoxify, causing inflammation and toxicity within your body. With daily dry brushing, you can increase oxygen flow, boost circulation, reduce appearance of cellulite, remove dead skin cells, and help your remaining cells and your body remove waste.

Dry brushing is extremely cleansing for your lymphatic system. Your lymphatic system is your body's natural detoxification system. It collects, transports, and eliminates the waste your cells produce. When your lymphatic system is congested, you experience toxic accumulation. Kapha types are most susceptible to congested lymphs, although everyone is susceptible, especially in the cold and wet Kapha months.

This is where dry brushing comes in. Dry brushing stimulates your lymphatic system and allows it to drain out the built-up toxicity within your bodies that naturally accumulates over time, especially if you're eating the wrong foods for your Dosha. Seasonal shifts, pesticides in foods, sugar, GMOs, and other factors increase toxins in your body, so it's recommended that you detoxify once a season.

Dry brushing should be practiced daily, both as a preventative measure to keep your lymphatic system operating strongly before it becomes congested and as a treatment for when you feel like your toxins have already accumulated. Dry brushing only takes 5 minutes a day to do, yet its benefits are infinite. Best of all, it's one of those things that feels just as good when you do it on yourself as when someone else does it on you—instant spa experience!

How to Dry Brush

If you've ever scrubbed your skin with a loofa, you actually already know how to dry brush. The process is quite similar, except you dry brush on dry skin, hence the name, to better remove dead, flaky skin cells.

You can use any natural, firm-bristle brush or purchase one specific for dry brushing. Strokes go toward your heart in long, slow motions.

Here's how to dry brush:

1. Begin on your arms, and using firm yet gentle strokes, stroke upward. Brush the various angles of your arms in long strokes, being sure not to press so hard that you break the skin, but not so soft that you aren't really doing anything. If you have rough, raised bumps on the back of your arms, focus on those spots.

2. After you've done both arms, move to your chest and stomach. These areas can be a little more sensitive, so use a lighter touch. Practice several long strokes, always toward your heart.

3. Move toward your back. If you have a lot of accumulated dead skin cells on your lower back (many of us do), this should be another area to target.

4. Head down to your feet, and perform several long strokes upward. Then dry brush all sides of your legs. This help reduce the appearance of cellulite, so pay particular attention to the back of your thighs and any other problem areas.

5. After dry brushing, either bathe or follow up with abhyanga, or self-oil massage.

You also can dry brush your face, which helps cleanse dirt, dead skin cells, and clogged pores. However, I recommend having a separate, softer, smaller brush for your face so you don't bring toxins from your body to your face.

Once a week, wash your brush in one cup warm water with 3 drops tea tree oil or neem. Lay the brush bristles down on a towel to allow to dry.

Abhyanga (Self-Oil Massage)

After you've sloughed away those dead skin cells, it's time to oil your body in a massaging practice called *abhyanga*. You don't have to go to a spa to get abhyanga done; you can practice it on yourself and still reap its wonderful benefits.

Just like dry brushing, abhyanga increases circulation, especially on nerve endings. Your skin is left dry and exposed after exfoliation, which is why it's healing to hydrate it with oil afterward. Oil is recommended over water-soluble creams and lotions because your skin absorbs it better and it doesn't contain any chemicals. Ayurveda states you shouldn't put anything on your skin you wouldn't eat; would you eat your chemical-laden lotions?

DEFINITION

Abhyanga is the ancient Ayurvedic practice of massaging your skin with oil to hydrate your body from within. It enhances muscle tone, detoxification, and relaxation.

Oil, especially when warmed, penetrates the deeper layers of your body, lubricating your joints and hydrating from within.

The Benefits of Abhyanga

Abhyanga has many benefits, including toning your muscles, enhancing detoxification, softening your skin, calming your nervous system, releasing fatigue, aiding your sleep, and improving elimination. You also can practice abhyanga in the morning, but I normally practice at night when I have more time and use it to help me drift off to sleep.

The Charaka Samhita states, "The body of one who uses oil massage regularly does not become affected much even if subjected to accidental injuries, or strenuous work. By using oil massage daily, a person is endowed with pleasant touch, trimmed body parts and becomes strong, charming and least affected by old age."

How to Practice Abhyanga

Practicing Abhyanga is very simple and quite intuitive. It's very similar to applying lotion, but more deliberate. The Sanskrit word for oil is *sneha*, which also means "love." When oiling your body, give love to yourself. Your body is your most prized possession, and you should treat it with the same love and care you would give a newborn baby.

In traditional Ayurvedic massage, the oil is warmed to make it more absorbable by the skin. You can warm the oil at home in a number of ways or even just rub it between your hands to warm it if you're pressed for time.

The touch of your self-massage depends on what you need and your Dosha. If you're feeling lethargic and heavy, like a Kapha, practice more vigorous, firm strokes to stimulate your body and get your muscles loosened. If you're stressed and tight, practice a slower and more deliberate massage. Always balance how your body is doing with your treatment.

Typically, you'll use between ¼ and ½ cup oil during your self-massage, depending on how dry your skin is, so have at least that amount available. I recommend purchasing organic, high-quality oil from an Ayurvedic herbal company, like those listed in Appendix B.

Here's how to practice abhyanga, self-oil massage:

1. First you must warm up the oil. There are three ways to do this.

2. The first way is to fill a glass bottle with the amount of oil you'd like to use and submerge it in a pot of hot water on the stove. The second way is to hold the glass bottle under hot running water until it is warm, which will take longer and also wastes water. The third way is to pour a tablespoon of oil in your palm and rub your palms in circular motions for 20 to 30 seconds, or until heat is generated between your hands

3. Create a small pool of warm oil in your hands and begin rubbing the oil into your arms. Pay particular attention to any dry spots on the back of your arms, on your elbows, and around your wrists.

4. Add more oil to your hands and begin gently massaging your abdomen in counterclockwise circular motions. This is the direction of your colon and the movement aids your digestion and elimination. Go up your right side, across your abdomen, and down your left side.

5. Bring the oil up to your chest in long, slow strokes toward your heart. This helps you connect with your heart chakra and emotions (more on chakras in Chapter 21).

6. Add more oil to your hands and massage your back, an area that holds a great deal of tension. It can be hard to reach your back, but try your best. Really massage the oil into your shoulders, lower back, and other areas where you hold tension.

7. Pour more oil into your hands and massage it into your buttocks and down your legs. You may notice that your skin absorbs a lot of oil in these areas.

8. Be sure to oil your feet as well, which are often dry and callused.

Put on socks after you oil your feet to retain the oil. When you're finished, put on pajamas that you don't mind getting a slight oil residue on as well.

 AYURVEDIC ALERT

> If you notice the oil is quickly disappearing as you apply it to certain spots (or all over), your skin is very dehydrated. You most likely have Vata skin, which is parched and dry. Frequently practicing abhyanga helps moisturize your skin from within.

You don't have to practice abhyanga every day. The recommended frequency depends on your Dosha:

Vatas: Practice at least five times a week. During cold, dry, Vata season, you may need to oil your body every day.

Pittas: Practice at least three times a week, using a cooling oil like coconut. You do not need to oil your body as much in the hot, humid months.

Kaphas: Practice at least two times a week if you're a Kapha because you naturally retain oil. Pay particular attention to the dry spots on your body, and add stimulating herbs to your oil. Sesame, almond, or olive oil are great choices for Kaphas.

I recommend oiling your scalp and giving yourself a head massage once a week. This enhances hair growth as well as calms the mind. If you have long hair, braid your hair and sleep overnight with the oil on your head. Place a towel over your pillow to keep it clean.

Some people practice abhyanga after a shower in place of using lotion, while others practice before showering so the oil can enter their skin during the shower. It's really your preference. I recommend that those who have drier skin or live somewhere with drier weather oil their bodies after their shower because the warm water dries the skin. If you're a Kapha type, are naturally oily, or just really dislike having oil on your body, you could practice abhyanga prior to bathing.

Types of Oils to Use

What types of oil you use for abhyanga depends on your Dosha type:

Vatas: Use a warming oil like sesame, which is considered the queen of oils. Be sure the oil is organic and untoasted. Almond oil is another good option because it's also warming. You could purchase herb-infused oils that have Vata-pacifying herbs within them as well.

Pittas: Use cooling oils, particularly coconut oil, which cools the body temperature and also heals redness and acne. Sunflower oil is also recommended for Pittas. You don't need to heat the oil.

Kaphas: Use warming oils, such as sesame or almond. Olive and corn oil are also good choices. You don't need as much oil as Vatas and Pittas.

Nasal Cleansing

Another Ayurvedic practice you could add to your nightly or morning routine is nasal cleansing. This is split into two practices: *neti* and *nasya*. Neti is the process of cleansing the nasal passages with salt water using a neti pot; nasya is the practice of lubricating the nasal cavities with oil. The two practices go hand in hand because one disinfects and then the other moisturizes and prevents the mucus from reforming.

> **DEFINITION**
>
> **Neti** and **nasya** are the Ayurvedic practices of cleansing the nasal passages. Neti is rinsing out the nostrils with salt water. Nasya is administering oil in the nostrils to heal allergies, improve breathing, relieve headaches, and even improve quality of voice.

Why Cleanse Your Nostrils?

You are constantly breathing in toxins, from pollution in the air to the fragrances in perfumes, air fresheners, and candles. As a result, your nasal passages become filled with toxicity and benefit from being cleaned out from time to time. All airborne illnesses begin in the nose, and when you clean your nostrils, you can prevent and heal allergies, colds, and flus.

Ayurveda states that nasal cleansing also is important because the nose is the direct route to the brain and the doorway to your consciousness. By cleansing your nasal passages, you improve your breathing; cure headaches; release tension; and overcome sinus infections, colds, flus, and allergies.

Neti

Neti pots come in ceramic, metal, and plastic, but it's best to avoid plastic. You can find neti pots in many stores, even supermarkets, and also online. (See Appendix B for some sources.)

Here's how to practice neti cleansing:

1. Thoroughly wash your neti pot to be sure it's clean.

2. In a pan, bring 1 or 2 cups water to boil to disinfect. Allow the water to cool to a warm temperature so you don't burn your nostrils. When the water is warm, pour it into your neti pot.

3. Add ¼ teaspoon sea salt per ½ cup warm water and stir

4. Stand over a sink, place the tip of the neti pot spout into your nostril, and tilt your head sideways without leaning your head forward or backward. The water should enter one nostril and flow out the other. Breathe through your mouth as you work. Use about half of the water in one nostril.

5. Repeat the process with the remaining water and your other nostril. Now your nasal passages are cleansed!

This practice kills bacteria and other debris that cause allergies and illness. You'll be amazed to see how quickly this practice clears up mucus.

Neti is not necessary for every day, but I highly recommend it during cold, flu, and allergy season. If you have a sinus infection or allergies, you can practice up to three times a day.

Nasya

Nasya is the practice of lubricating the nasal passages with oil, and it's best performed after neti cleansing. The salt water from neti can dry out your nasal passages, which stimulates your body to secrete more mucus to protect the membranes. Nasya lubricates those membranes with oil so your body doesn't create more mucus. It's a wonderful preventative measure to overcome a stuffy nose and is the reason why saline solution alone is not enough; you need both salt water and oil together.

Nasya is said to improve the quality of your voice, improve your vision, promote mental clarity, release tension headaches, heal sinus congestion, and release stress.

Nasya oil is a specific type of medicated oil typically comprised of sesame oil and medicinal herbs. You can find nasya oil on many Ayurvedic websites. If you can't find it, you can use sesame oil.

There are two ways you can practice nasya. In the first way, which is the most effective, you lie down on your back and administer the oil in your nose. You'll eventually get used to it, but at first it might feel weird to have oil go up your nose.

> **WISDOM OF THE AGES**
>
> At my first Ayurvedic treatment in India, I was shocked when the practitioner suddenly squirted oil up my nose mid-massage. It felt like I had just inhaled water while swimming. When you practice nasya on yourself, you have more control and will be prepared for the oily splash.

If you'd like to go this route, here's how:

1. Lie down on your back, preferably on your bed.

2. Tilt your head backward, either off the edge of the bed or by placing a pillow below your middle back so your head is leaning backward.

3. With a dropper, release 5 to 10 drops of room temperature nasya oil in each nostril.

4. Inhale deeply and lie still for a few minutes so the nasya oil can deeply penetrate your nasal passages. It will feel a bit strange at the beginning, but it's definitely worth the benefits.

The second way is to put a drop of nasya oil on your pinky finger and insert it into your nostril. You won't be able to get as deep as you would when you're lying down, but it will still lubricate your nostril's inner walls and is a great starting point.

The Least You Need to Know

- Prepare your body for sleep by diffusing sleep-inducing essential oils or burning soy candles. Avoid paraffin and artificially scented candles, air fresheners, fragranced sprays, and incense.
- Dry brush away the dead layers of your skin with a firm-bristled brush to remove toxins and stimulate your lymphatic system.
- Oil your body with organic, unprocessed oil specific to your Dosha to hydrate and soften your skin.
- If you have allergies or a sinus infection, cleanse your nose with a neti pot and lubricate it with nasya oil.

Ayurvedic Nutrition

As a Certified Ayurvedic, Holistic, and Sports Nutritionist, this section is really my forte. In these chapters, I give you all the information you need to know about Ayurvedic food and eating. I discuss the digestive fire, the Ayurvedic diet philosophy, common nutritional disorders and food toxins to be aware of, and my favorite, delicious recipes you can try to begin eating Ayurvedically.

CHAPTER 12

The Digestive Fire Agni

Inside of every person is a bright fire, called their *agni*. It governs digestion, metabolism, and nutrient assimilation and absorption. Essentially, your fire is the key to your health. When your fire is burning brightly, you can digest your food and reap its benefits. When your fire is depleted, toxins begin accumulating in your body.

In this chapter, I explain the importance of this internal flame that keeps your body alive. I also share the four types of agni—balanced, irregular, sharp, and dull—so you can see how your digestive system stacks up.

In This Chapter

- Agni, your fire within
- Qualities of balanced and imbalanced agni
- What Dosha is your digestion?
- Eating for your digestive type

Understanding Agni

Put your hands on your belly and breathe for a few moments. You are touching the most powerful part of your body, which takes your food and turns it into energy, nutrients, muscle tissues, blood, organs, and so much more. This robust part of your body is your agni, your digestive fire.

In Ayurveda, it's said that a man is only as old as his agni. If he digests food well, he will never age. But the moment your digestive system starts to falter, you begin aging and accumulating disease. This is why a healthy digestion is the cornerstone of health.

> **DEFINITION**
>
> **Agni** is your internal fire, in charge of digestion, nutrient assimilation, metabolism, and creation of bodily tissues. It's hot, sharp, light, mobile, dry, and subtle, most similar to the Pitta Dosha and most different from the Kapha Dosha. When your agni is healthy, you can easily digest both foods and emotions, making you physically and mentally sound. When your agni is too much or too little, you begin suffering from digestive, health, and emotional issues.

The Importance of Your Internal Fire

Think of your agni like the process of cooking a dish. When you open your mouth, you put all the raw ingredients into the pot to be cooked. If your fire is strong, the food will be cooked in no time. If your fire is too strong, the food will burn. If your fire is too weak, the food will remain raw. This is how your digestive fire works.

All plant-based ingredients contain nutrients available for your body to take in and use. However, if you aren't properly cooking those foods in your body, they don't do you any good. This undigested food begins to rot in your gastrointestinal tract, and over time, this rotting begins to ferment, spreading toxicity throughout your body. You experience these toxins through bad breath, a white coating on your tongue, acne, and other imbalances.

If you experience bloating, gas, constipation, diarrhea, heartburn or acid reflux, indigestion, water retention, heaviness or lethargy after meals, or weight gain, your digestive fire is not burning at optimal strength.

Digestion and the Doshas

Bloating, gas, and constipation are symptoms of Vata. Diarrhea, heartburn/acid reflux, and indigestion are signs of Pitta. Water retention, heaviness/lethargy, and weight gain are signs of Kapha.

Vata is an airy energy, so you begin experiencing symptoms of excess airiness in your digestive system, leading to bloating and gas. It's also a cold and dry energy, attributing to hard, dry stools and constipation.

Pitta is a fiery energy, and agni is also fire. What happens when fire meets fire? Chaos. Diarrhea, heartburn/acid reflux, and indigestion occur when the fire in your body is too strong. Your body produces acid to break down food, but if you have too much acid, you'll experience heartburn and acid reflux. Similarly, when food passes through your system too quickly, you don't receive its nutrients, resulting in watery stool. Indigestion occurs when your digestion is too sharp, causing pain.

Kapha is an earthy energy, making you extremely grounded. Too much of this can make you heavy like the soil though. Kapha types tend to retain water, causing further heaviness. If the digestive system is dull, then you cannot utilize those calories as energy, attributing to weight gain. If you've ever felt exhausted after a meal, this was an increase in Kapha energy.

 AYURVEDIC ALERT

Feeling bloated, gassy, and constipated? Vata's wind has picked up in your colon. Running to the bathroom after meals or experiencing heartburn, acid reflux, or indigestion? Gotta put out that Pitta fire. Does a single meal make you feel like you've gained 10 pounds and want to hibernate? That means Kapha is on the loose.

Your Body Begins with Digestion

Once your food is digested, it turns into your physical body. A healthy agni can take a piece of raw material, food, and turn it into your liver, kidneys, skin, and blood. An unhealthy agni won't be able to nourish these parts of your body to the level they need, resulting in disease.

Agni influences the following bodily functions:

Darshana: Promotes eye health

Matroshna: Regulates body temperature

Prakruti varna: Maintains *(agni)* skin color

Dhatu poshanam: Promotes bodily tissue health

Ojah kara: Production of *ojas,* immune system maintenance

Tejah kara: Production of *tejas,* maintenance of cell membranes and semipermeability of capillaries

Pranakara: Production of *prana* life force, maintenance of breath and life

Dirgham: Lifespan maintenance

Prabha: Maintenance of healthy skin glow and luster

Bala: Provides strength, energy, and vitality

So what happens when agni goes sour? Quite simply, you experience imbalances in the preceding areas.

Adarshanam: Impaired vision, glaucoma, cataracts, iritis, corneal opacity

Amatroshna: Hypothermia (decreased body temperature) or pyrexia (increased body temperature)

Vikruti varna: Abnormal skin color (If you have excess Vata, you'll have dark pigmentation. If you have excess Pitta, you'll have yellow or red discoloration. If you have excess Kapha, you'll have extreme paleness.)

Dhatu karshyana: Tissue emaciation if agni too high; unprocessed bodily tissues if agni is too low

Ojohara: Diminished immunity, leading to autoimmune disorders

Tejohara: Decreased cell permeability, leading to decreased nutrient and mineral absorption

Pranahara: Weak life force, low energy, poor breathing

Imbalanced *dirgham:* Early death, loss of zest for life

Chaya: Unhealthy complexion

Kshaya: Decayed strength

Constipation, diarrhea, bloating, heartburn, and lethargy are more than just temporary grievances you have to deal with. They are signals that deeper components of your health are not functioning. It's extremely important that you consume foods that are easy to digest because your agni is in charge of every function in your body and also your mind. Without healthy agni, your physical and mental health will deteriorate.

Your Second Brain

Agni controls more than just your physical digestion. It also helps you digest emotions. Have you ever heard someone say, "That person is so constipated." Surely, they weren't talking about their bowels! A "constipated" person is one who is tense and stuck, sort of like constipated stool.

The state of your digestion affects your mind. In fact, *Scientific American* reported that research has found that 95 percent of your serotonin is found in your bowels. For that reason, your gut is literally your second brain. This second brain contains 100 million neurons, which is more than you have in your spinal cord or peripheral nervous system.

Agni has several emotional functions listed in Ayurveda:

Shauryam: Confidence, courage, bravery

Harshna: Joy, cheerfulness, laughter, happiness

Dhariyam: Patience, stability, balance

Medhakara: Intelligence, cellular communication

Buddhikara: Logic, mental reasoning, discrimination

Prasada: Mental clarity, comprehension, consistency

Raga: Enthusiasm, interest, affection, colorful personality

Ayurveda knew back then, without any scientific evidence, that digestion also controls mental health. Research today confirms this finding and even has linked autism, attention-deficit/hyperactivity disorder (ADHD), and other mental disorders to poor digestion.

When agni is imbalanced, you experience the opposite of the emotional functions listed earlier:

Ashauryam: Fear, anxiety (Vata related)

Aharshna: Depression, sadness (Kapha related)

Adhirata: Impatience (Pitta related) or sloppiness (Kapha related)

Medhahara: Lack of cellular communication causing illness, including cancer (can be related to any Dosha)

Buddhihara: Indecisiveness (Vata related)

Vishada: Confusion, scatter-mindedness, inconsistency (Vata related)

Viraga: Withdrawal, depression (Kapha related)

Which of these relate to you?

WISDOM OF THE AGES

A healthy gut means a healthy mind. When your digestion is working well, you experience confidence, joy, patience, logic, mental clarity, and enthusiasm. When it's off balance, you might suffer from anxiety, depression, impatience, indecisiveness, confusion, withdrawal, or disease, depending on your Doshic constitution.

The Four Types of Digestive Fires

Now that you know the physical and mental symptoms of an imbalanced agni, let's figure out which Dosha your digestion is. As mentioned earlier, the various qualities are related to specific Doshas. We all are susceptible to specific digestive imbalances depending on our Doshic constitution:

Vata Vikruti: Cold, dry, and irregular digestive system.

Pitta Vikruti: Hot, sharp, and acidic digestive system.

Kapha Vikruti: Slow, heavy, and weak digestive system.

It's also possible to have no negative digestive side effects. That's when your Doshas are balanced.

Ayurveda classifies these four varieties as *sama agni* (balanced), *vishama agni* (Vata), *tikshna agni* (Pitta), and *manda agni* (Kapha). Each of these digestive types has its own mental and physical imbalances. Let's figure out yours with this quick quiz:

1. How do you feel after a meal?

    a. Good, energized

    b. Depends what I ate, often bloated or gassy

    c. Usually good but sometimes suffer from heartburn if I ate the wrong foods

    d. Heavy, stuffed, and exhausted

2. How often are you hungry?

    a. Pretty regularly

    b. Varies every day

    c. Almost always

    d. Rarely; I stay full for a long time

3. How is your stool?

    a. Normal

    b. Usually dry and small but sometimes diarrhea

    c. Frequent, sometimes liquidy

    d. Heavy, dense

4. Which foods tend to bother you the most?

    a. I'm pretty good with most foods

    b. Cauliflower, broccoli, any cruciferous vegetable

    c. Fried or spicy foods, garlic, tomatoes

    d. Sweets, carbs, heavy foods

Now count how many a, b, c, and d answers you got.

If you scored mostly a answers, you have sama agni, which is a balanced digestive system. If you scored mostly b answers, you have vishama agni, which is a Vata digestive system. If you scored mostly c answers, you have tikshna agni, which is a Pitta digestive system. If you scored mostly d answers, you have manda agni, which is a Kapha digestive system.

WISDOM OF THE AGES

Sama agni means the digestive fire is balanced with no issues. Vishama agni means there is excess Vata in the digestive fire, causing issues such as gas and bloating. Tikshna agni means there is excess Pitta in the digestive fire, causing acidity and constant hunger. Manda agni means there is excess Kapha in the digestive system, leading to sluggish metabolism and weight gain.

Sama Agni (Balanced)

Those with sama agni are the lucky ones who have achieved balance. They feel energized after a meal, not stuffed or exhausted. They even can eat ingredients not in season or not follow food-combining rules and still be fine. They have strong immune systems and reap the nutrients from the foods they eat. Their appetites are regular and stable, they feel hunger at mealtimes, and they have the ability to stop eating when they're full.

Mentally, they are peaceful, vibrant, and loving.

These are the benefits of a healthy digestive system.

Vishama Agni (Vata, Irregular)

Those with vishama agni have many of symptoms of Vata. Their digestive system is irregular, just like the Vata wind. Some days they have never-ending appetites, and other days they just aren't hungry at all. Similarly, their digestive fire is cold and weak, leaving them extremely bloated after meals. Gas forms in their colons easily, and they often suffer from constipation.

Mentally, they may experience Vata side effects like anxiety, insecurity, overanalyzing, and insomnia. This cold and dry digestive fire leads to Vata imbalances within the body, including dry skin, cracking joints, back pain, and other Vata side effects. It is important that they warm up and lubricate their digestive fires to regain balance.

Tikshna Agni (Pitta, Sharp)

People with tikshna agni have sharp and fiery digestive fires, just like Pitta. They have rampant appetites and become angry when they miss a meal. They often can get away with eating whatever they want, which causes them to eat the wrong types of food. They then may suffer from heartburn and hyperacidity. Their digestive fires are too hot, and food may move straight through their systems, resulting in loose stool.

Mentally, those with tikshna agni may experience Pitta side effects, including impatience, irritability, anger, and resentment. They are staunch perfectionists and may become obsessive. They also may experience Pitta side effects, including nausea, inflammation, and hot flashes. It's essential that they cool down their sharp digestive fires to reach sama agni.

Manda Agni (Kapha, Dull)

Manda agni causes a slow, heavy, and cool digestive fire. Sufferers gain weight after almost anything they eat. At the same time, they don't eat much. Their metabolisms are just so slow that whatever they do eat causes them to gain weight. They often aren't hungry in the morning but still feel heavy and dull.

Mentally, those with manda agni may feel lazy, exhausted, or cloudy. After eating, instead of feeling energized, they feel lethargic and cannot move or focus. They may experience other Kapha side effects such as depression, attachment, emotional eating, and cold and clammy skin. It's best they consume a well-spiced and hot diet to reignite their dull digestive fires.

 AYURVEDIC ALERT

Are you a big fan of ice-cream? Unfortunately, that's the number one thing that causes manda agni in Ayurveda. It is cold, heavy and full of dairy, all things that imbalance Kapha, causing weight-gain and lethargy. Though giving up ice-cream may seem impossible, you'll feel so much better when it's not in your system.

The following table compares the physical and mental symptoms of the various agni types and the Dosha they are related to.

The Four Agni Types

Agni Type	Related Dosha	Physical Symptoms	Mental Symptoms
Sama agni	All	Strong digestion, stable appetite, healthy immune system	Energized after meals, clear and loving mind
Vishama agni	Vata	Irregular appetite, gas, constipation, dry body	Anxiety, insecurity, fear, insomnia
Tikshna agni	Pitta	Large appetite, loose stools, hyperacidity	Anger, impatience
Manda agni	Kapha	Poor digestion, gains weight easily, loss of appetite	Sleepy, tired, weakness

The Best Foods for Each Agni Type

Food is medicine. You can heal your body just by changing your diet. As discussed, all parts of your body begin in your gut, including your physical and mental well-being. By following the right diet for your unique digestive fire, you can treat and prevent many of the imbalances outlined earlier.

Foods for Vishama Agni

If you have many of the symptoms of vishama agni, you'll want to follow a Vata-pacifying diet. That means staying away from cold, raw, and dry foods and consuming more warm, cooked, grounding foods.

Foods to eat more of:

- All types of nuts and seeds
- Mung beans
- Roasted vegetable soups, stews, and curries
- Root vegetables, particularly ginger, yams, and squash
- Sesame oil
- Sweet fruit
- Warming grains

These Vata-pacifying foods enhance your digestive fire and are easy to digest, bringing you back to sama agni.

Foods to stay away from:

- Chips
- Crackers
- Granola bars
- Iced water, coffee, tea, or soda

- Popcorn
- Salads
- Smoothies

These foods further extinguish your already-weak digestive fire. Instead, you must warm it up and create moisture from within. A dehydrated colon leads to constipation, which is why it's best to drink warm water frequently and add warming oils to your diet.

Foods for Tikshna Agni

If you have many of the symptoms of tikshna agni, you'll want to follow a Pitta-pacifying diet. That means staying away from spicy, oily, and fried foods, as well as stimulants like caffeine and chocolate. Instead, focus on cooling and cleansing ingredients.

Foods to eat more of:

- All legumes
- Coconut oil
- Cooling grains
- Cruciferous vegetables

- Fresh fruit
- Greens
- Herbs
- Seeds

These Pitta-pacifying ingredients cool your aggravated digestive fire, allowing you to regain sama agni.

Foods to stay away from:

- Chiles
- Chocolate
- Coffee
- Fried foods and tempuras
- Garlic and onions

- Nuts
- Oily curries, stews, or stir-fries
- Tomatoes and all nightshade vegetables

These foods disrupt your already irritated digestive fire, causing your symptoms to become worse. Focus on cooling your body and cleansing it with hydrating foods. Avoid nightshade vegetables and garlic, which are very pungent and also disrupt Pitta.

> **WISDOM OF THE AGES**
>
> Nightshade vegetables are part of the Solanaceae plant family and contain alkaloids to defend themselves from insects at night. These alkaloids are particularly disruptive for Pitta types. Nightshades include tomatoes, eggplant, peppers, chiles, and potatoes.

Foods for Manda Agni

If you have many of the symptoms of manda agni, you are best following a Kapha-pacifying diet. This includes avoiding heavy, sweet, starchy, and fattening foods, which will make you feel more exhausted and cause you to gain more weight. To shed those pounds and regain energy, eat a diet that is well spiced and vibrant.

Foods to eat more of:

- All types of spices
- Blended vegetable soups
- Cruciferous vegetables
- Legumes
- Low-sugar fruit
- Seeds
- Small amounts of grains and oils
- Steamed bitter vegetables, including leafy greens, brussels sprouts, and asparagus

These Kapha-pacifying ingredients are easy to digest and stimulate your digestive fire, helping you regain sama agni.

Foods to stay away from:

- Dairy products
- Fried foods
- Starches, including bread, pasta, and excess rice
- Sugar, maple syrup, honey and other forms of sugar
- Sweet fruit, including dates, bananas, mangoes and dried fruit

These foods make you feel heavier and more lethargic, attributing to weak digestion and weight gain. Stimulate your body through your diet with light, well-spiced, and easily digested meals. Cook vegetables slightly to make them easier to digest.

> **WISDOM OF THE AGES**
>
> Having manda agni doesn't mean you have to avoid all sweet things forever. Monkfruit and stevia are two types of natural sweeteners that have no impact on your blood sugar levels, making them a great option for Kapha types, those seeking to lose weight, diabetics, and those with manda agni digestive systems.

The Least You Need to Know

- Your digestion is referred to as your agni because it is a fire within your body, cooking your food and turning it into nutrients.
- Digestion plays a role not only in your body, but also in your mind, causing everything from indecisiveness to depression.
- There are four types of agni: sama, vishama, tikshna, and manda.
- Sama agni means balanced. Vishama agni is Vata-imbalanced. Tikshna agni is Pitta-imbalanced. Manda agni is Kapha-imbalanced.
- To regain sama agni, or a balanced digestive fire, you must follow a diet to pacify the imbalanced Dosha. That means more cooked and warming foods for vishama agni, more hydrating and cooling foods for tikshna agni, and more light and stimulating foods for manda agni.

CHAPTER 13

The Ayurvedic Perspective on Nutrition

More people are aware of the herbal and skin-care sides of Ayurveda than with its nutritional theories. As an Ayurvedic nutritionist, I have found so much intuitive wisdom in the way Ayurveda explains nutrition, illustrating the connection between someone's everyday diet and later illnesses.

The Ayurvedic perspective of nutrition is all about balance. Ayurveda is less concerned with calories and macronutrients and more concerned with energy and maintaining equilibrium. When you are eating the right diet in the right amounts, you will be consuming the calories and nutrients you need effortlessly, without even needing to worry about them.

In this chapter, I review the five types of nutritional disorders according to Ayurveda. Most likely, you or someone close to you suffers from at least one. These disorders are much more common than you'd believe and are the leading causes of digestive issues and chronic disease. After explaining these disorders, I explain how to treat and prevent each through dietary and lifestyle practices you can begin implementing today. With proper nutrition, you can become your healthiest self, one bite at a time.

In This Chapter

- Nutritional disorders according to Ayurveda
- The health effects of overeating and undereating
- Why we need to stop eating leftovers
- The real reason so many of us are overweight
- Ways to heal your body with food

The Five Types of Nutritional Disorders

When you think of nutritional disorders, you might think of malnourishment on one end of the scale and obesity on the other. The many types of nutritional disorders that lie in between these two extremes frequently are overlooked.

Many of us suffer from nutritional disorders without having any idea. We believe we are healthy but little things we are doing like eating too much at dinner, buying snacks from the convenient store, and even having leftovers can lead to a nutritional disorder.

Ayurveda classifies five main types of nutritional disorders:

- Quantitative dietary deficiency
- Qualitative dietary deficiency
- Quantitative and qualitative overnutrition
- Toxins in food
- Foods unstable for one's Doshic constitution

Let's take a closer view of each.

Quantitative Dietary Deficiency

Quantitative dietary deficiencies are caused by not eating the right amount of food. This includes malnourishment, starvation, anorexia, and excess fasting. Quantitative dietary deficiencies are more common in the developing world, where food sources are scarce, but they are on the rise in developed countries with the progression of eating disorders, particularly in young women.

Qualitative Dietary Deficiency

Qualitative dietary deficiencies result from not eating enough nutritionally sound food. This is another type of malnourishment, yet it stems from not consuming enough nutrients even though you might be consuming enough calories. Qualitative dietary deficiency is much more common than you'd think. Eating too many processed, packaged, and precooked foods causes qualitative dietary deficiency. Improper food combining can lead to this type of deficiency as well. Most Americans have this deficiency and don't even know it.

Quantitative and Qualitative Overnutrition

This is another deficiency a huge percentage of the population suffers from: eating too much food. In fact, two thirds of Americans are overweight. Overnutrition results in obesity, diabetes, high cholesterol, lethargy, cold sweats, heart disease, and stroke. Emotional, binge, and mindless eating, as well as overeating all cause quantitative and qualitative overnutrition.

Toxins in Food

Unless you live on an organic farm and grow your own food, you most likely have some level of this disorder. Genetically modified foods, pesticides, hormones, and antibiotics in many of our food ingredients can lead to toxicity, attributing to digestive disorders and other illnesses. You can minimize this disorder by consuming an organic, diet free of genetically modified foods.

Foods Unstable for One's Doshic Constitution

Before you read this book, you may have been eating the wrong foods for your Dosha every day and not even realized it. When you eat the wrong foods for your Doshic constitution, imbalances accumulate, from acne to arthritis. Your digestion is the cornerstone of your health, which is why you must eat the right foods for your Dosha.

> **AYURVEDIC ALERT**
>
> Nutritional disorders stem from undereating, overeating, consuming nutrient-void foods (packaged, processed, precooked), toxicity in foods (pesticides, GMOs, antibiotics, hormones), and eating the wrong ingredients for your Doshic constitution. You might be suffering from one or more of these and not necessarily know it.

Treating the Disorders

As you can see, these nutritional deficiencies are much more common than you might have imagined. But hope is not lost; they all are treatable and preventable.

According to Ayurveda, true health comes in your everyday actions. You don't need to take an array of vitamins and supplements to be healthy. Health comes from your food. Your vegetables are your vitamin shots. Your spices are your medicine. Your fruits are your beauty pills. You don't need to look for health anywhere else besides your plate.

Just as important as *what* you eat is *how* you eat. If you consume too much or too little food, you'll experience a nutritional disorder. At the same time, if you eat for reasons other than hunger—such as anger, loneliness, sadness, or boredom—you're setting yourself up for disaster.

Food is much more than something you mindlessly put in your mouth to survive; it is energy, ritual, medicine, community, and joy. By healing your relationship with food, you can heal your body.

Quantitative Deficiencies

It's hard to believe anyone would intentionally not eat enough food to nourish and sustain their body, but that's what happens with quantitative dietary deficiencies.

A Closer Look at Quantitative Deficiencies

Although you live in the Western world where food is abundant, more and more people are suffering from quantitative nutritional deficiencies, meaning they are malnourishing themselves by choice. Why is it when the grocery stores are full of food, people are purposely going hungry? Because they've been told by the media that women are more desirable the thinner they are.

The Western fashion industry has glorified Vata-imbalanced bodies, with visible collarbones, protruding hips, "thigh gaps," and tiny figures. However, in many other parts of the world, it is actually more desirable for women to have some extra body fat because it signifies her fertility and health. In fact, in India, men are encouraged to marry Kapha women because they are best suited as wives—peaceful, motherly, fertile, and strong. (It is interesting to note how each society has its own unique version of beauty and observe how your own view has been influenced by your surroundings.)

Regardless of cultural trends, you must find the right weight for your unique body type. Each Dosha has its own physiology: Vatas are naturally leaner, Pittas are more muscular, and Kaphas are curvier. Even if everyone followed the same diet and exercise routine, they would not all weigh the same amount because they each have a unique Prakriti. Many Kapha types particularly undereat to achieve this more Vata-esque body, which leads to a quantitative deficiency.

A woman who has a quantitative disorder constantly feels cold and sometimes even grows body hair to keep her warm. She may suffer from digestive issues, especially bloating, gas, and constipation, due to a low digestive fire. She may have visible bones, aching and cracking joints, and back pain. Her skin will have lost its vibrancy, and her hair will begin to shed. She may stop menstruating all together, a disorder called secondary amenorrhea. Her sex drive will decrease, as will her fertility, because her body is not in a healthy-enough state to reproduce.

Quantitative deficiency results in a Vata Vikruti, meaning one's Vata levels will increase out of balance.

Treating Quantitative Deficiencies

If this sounds like you or someone you know, following a Vata-pacifying diet and lifestyle is essential. Here are some tips to treat a quantitative dietary deficiency:

- Add more cooked foods to your diet.

- Eat more soups, curries, stews, and stir-fries.

- Include grains in all meals.

- Consume more root vegetables, particularly yams and squash.

- Incorporate warming spices in your diet, particularly ginger and cumin.

- Include more healthy fats in your diet, such as oils, nuts, and avocados.

- Avoid raw and cold foods, including salads, smoothies, popcorn, and crackers.

- Say no to iced drinks, such as iced water, coffee, or tea.

- Keep your body warm, staying away from the cold and wind.

- Be careful not to overwork your body, through overexercise or excess activity.

Continue following these suggestions until your weight has gone up and your body has regained balance.

Qualitative Deficiencies

Another type of malnourishment that's even more common is qualitative deficiency. This occurs when you eat enough calories but they're far from sufficiently nourishing.

A Closer Look at Qualitative Deficiencies

Empty calories are a big cause of qualitative deficiency. Consuming junk, processed food, and fat foods most certainly leads to this type of disorder. Many Americans consume frozen dinners, snacks from the vending machine, and premade foods. According to Ayurveda, this is all toxic. You must consume freshly cooked vegetables, grains, and legumes to receive the nutrients you need.

Ayurveda highly emphasizes the importance of fresh food. Never consume food that was made more than 24 hours ago, including your own leftovers. This is because the *prana,* or life force, of food depletes after it has been cooked. Therefore, if you consume food prepared more than a day ago, its nutritional content has diminished.

Reheating foods, especially in the microwave, further kills the food's remaining prana, making it nutritionally void. Food that no longer has nutritional value is more difficult for your body to digest. When your food is not well digested, toxins begin accumulating in your body, making you susceptible to imbalances. The fresher your food, the more healing benefits it offers your body.

> **WISDOM OF THE AGES**
>
> Enjoy your meal immediately after preparing it. Food begins to lose key nutrients as soon as you chop and cook it, and after 24 hours, it's nearly nutritionally void. Instead of eating yesterday's leftovers or heating a frozen dinner, make a meal from scratch.

Improper food combining can lead to a qualitative dietary deficiency as well. Ayurveda recommends specific rules of eating to prevent improper digestion, yet many of these rules are commonly broken, including these:

- Never eat starches (bread, rice, pasta) with animal proteins (chicken, beef, fish, etc.). This means a sandwich or chicken and rice is not correct food combining.

- Always eat fruit on an empty stomach, on its own, before meals.

- Never consume dairy products with fruit such as a milkshake or fruit parfait.

By breaking these food-combining rules, you set yourself up for digestive disasters, including heartburn, indigestion, bloating, diarrhea, constipation, and other issues that can further manifest as imbalances throughout your body.

Treating Qualitative Dietary Deficiencies

If you eat a lot of packaged, precooked, or processed foods, you likely suffer from a qualitative dietary deficiency. Most restaurants do not pay attention to food combining and add salt, unhealthy oils, and other ingredients to make their food tasty and affordable but not necessarily nutritious. Your health is not a priority as much as their profit.

Although it might seem difficult to not reheat yesterday's leftovers, especially if you made too much, the trick is to just prepare what you will eat that day. Most of us overshop and overcook. By frequently buying small amounts of local foods and cooking only what you will eat, you prevent qualitative nutritional deficiencies, resulting in increased energy, enhanced digestion, more vibrant skin, and a healthy physique.

Here are some tips to prevent a qualitative dietary deficiency:

- Eat something green every day, whether that's spinach, asparagus, broccoli, or anything in between. Green M&M's don't count.

- Shop at your local farmers' market to ensure you get the freshest food.

- Purchase only what you will eat for the next few days, and go back when you need more. I recommend grocery shopping twice a week.

- Buy a rice cooker to easily prepare rice, stews, and other dishes in a short amount of time with little effort.

- Try one-pot recipes like stews, curries, and stir-fries to lessen cleanup.

- Cook what you will eat that day. This prevents you from making excess food and overeating because you don't want to waste it.

Quantitative and Qualitative Overnutrition

Quantitative and qualitative overnutrition is the reason so many people are overweight or obese. In fact, it's the most common of them all.

A Closer Look at Quantitative and Qualitative Overnutrition

We've all been guilty of eating more than we're supposed to at least once or twice. But for many of us, it's once or twice *a day*. According to the National Institute of Diabetes and Digestive and Kidney Diseases (NIDDK), 68.6 percent of adults are considered overweight or obese, meaning their body mass index (BMI) is above 25. That's two thirds of the population. On top of that, one in three adults in the United States is considered obese, with a BMI above 30.

BMI is a measure of body fat based on height and weight. It's not a perfect indicator of your health because it doesn't differentiate between muscle and fat, but it does give you an overall indicator of your health. If you don't know your BMI, any number of online calculators can help you determine it.

To put these BMI measurements into more common terms, an average-build woman who is 5 feet, 5 inches tall would have to weigh 150 pounds to be considered overweight and 180 pounds to be considered obese. An average-build man 5 feet, 9 inches tall would have to weigh 170 pounds to be considered overweight and 203 pounds to be considered obese.

Food is energy. When you consume too much and don't burn it off, that energy has nowhere to go and is stored as fat. Once it's stored as fat, it's much more difficult to use than when it's still in food form, ready to be burned off. This is why exercise is vital for weight management. You can't keep putting fuel in your body without putting mileage on it to burn that fuel.

Overeating often stems from your culture. You are constantly busy and eating on the go, not allowing yourselves time to sit down and enjoy your meals. This continual state of stress makes you use food as a crutch or source of entertainment. Your restaurant portions are more than double the size of what you need, and your schools, offices, and even hospitals are bombarded with cookies, candy, and donuts. Eating has become America's favorite pastime, resulting in overnutrition.

> **WISDOM OF THE AGES**
>
> People often eat for emotional reasons, not necessarily because they're hungry. Emotional eating is on the rise as people use food as a coping mechanism for stress, loneliness, boredom, or unhappiness. Or they use food as a reward after a tough day at work and think they "deserve" a good binge because of the struggles they faced that day. Food temporarily takes your mind off your stress, but the moment you finish eating, you feel even worse, perpetuating the cycle. The only way to combat overnutrition is through self-love. When you care about yourself, you are less likely to overeat. You treat your body with the utmost care and become more in touch with what it actually needs.

Treating Quantitative and Qualitative Overnutrition

Quantitative and qualitative overnutrition causes Kapha imbalances, contributing to weight gain, diabetes, obesity, laziness, lethargy, heaviness, cold sweats, and depression.

Here are some tips to reverse quantitative and qualitative overnutrition:

- Drink warm water throughout the day. This increases your metabolism by 30 percent.

- Set your portions. Never eat out of a big bowl or container. Set a plate for yourself, and mindfully stick it.

- Eat slower, let your food linger, and chew well. Notice the tastes and textures of your food, and make eating an experience. Take at least 30 minutes to eat a meal.

- Do not eat while watching television, in front of your laptop, or on a mobile device. Focus on your food.

- Cook your own meals. You rarely know what's really in the food you buy in restaurants because it's often packed with salt, sugar, and unhealthy oils. When you cook your own food, you can control what you put in your body.

- Say no to dessert. Sip on ginger tea instead to stimulate your digestive fire. Sugar is an addictive substance that will keep this disorder going.

- Get moving. Sweat for at least 30 minutes a day to boost your metabolism. The best time to exercise is in the morning.

- After meals, don't collapse on the couch but instead walk for at least 15 minutes to promote digestion.

- Eat two or three meals a day, and avoid snacking in between. It is only between digestion periods that your body can detoxify. If you are constantly eating, you miss out on this detoxification.

- Practice self-care. The more you care for your body, the more you will want to treat it well.

- Give yourself an oil massage, dry brush your skin, make a facial mask, and perform all the other Ayurvedic acts of self-care. These practices teach you to value your body.

Toxins in Food

As you bite into a seemingly safe shiny apple or piece of moist and juicy chicken, you may be unaware of the pesticides, antibiotics, hormones, and other toxins the food contains. Ayurveda states that toxicity in our food is a leading cause of nutritional disorders. Although toxins came from bacteria 5,000 years ago, today they result from the antibiotics and pesticides used to treat them.

Some of the most common, and dangerous, toxins in our foods are pesticides, recombinant bovine growth hormone (rBGH), genetically modified organisms (GMOs), artificial food coloring and dyes, sodium nitrite/nitrate, bisphenol A (BPA), sodium aluminum sulphate, and potassium aluminum sulphate.

Let's look at the implications of the first three.

Pesticides

Pesticides are used to control and prevent pests such as insects, rodents, weeds, bacteria, mold, and fungi from damaging food. After it's applied, pesticide residue remains on your food and has been linked to cancer, birth defects, asthma, hormone disruption, and neurotoxicity. The toxic insecticide produced by genetically modified corn, for example, has been found in the blood of pregnant women and their unborn fetuses.

Ayurveda recommends consuming organic foods to avoid chemical exposure to potentially dangerous pesticides.

Recombinant Bovine Growth Hormone

rBGH is a synthetic, manmade hormone given to dairy cows to increase milk production. It's illegal in the European Union, Canada, and other countries due to its potential health effects, but it's been approved by the U.S. Food and Drug Administration since 1993. Many medical health experts have declared rBGH unsafe, including Samuel Epstein, MD, in his book *What's in Your Milk?*

Drinking milk from cows treated with rBGH increases blood levels of the growth hormone insulin-like growth factor 1 (IGF-1). The American Cancer Society reports early studies linking IGF-1 to tumor development, particularly in breast, prostate, and colorectal cancer.

Cows treated with rBGH are more likely to develop udder infections, called mastitis, leading to bacteria and pus in milk. This problem is what caused the European Union and other countries to ban rBGH. The United States deals with this issue by feeding cows antibiotics, which leads to more antibiotic-resistant bacteria and also may kill our own healthy gut bacteria when we consume the antibiotic-laden dairy products.

In Ayurvedic times, people drank milk from their neighborhood cow and ate plants from their garden, which happened to be organic, raw, non-GMO, and rBGH free. Today, we have to pay attention and seek out safe products to ensure our foods are toxin free.

Genetically Modified Organisms

GMOs are plants, animals, or other organisms whose genetic makeups have been modified using recombinant DNA methods, gene modification, or transgenic technology. Since GMOs were introduced in 1996, chronic illnesses, food allergies, and other disorders have been on the rise. The percentage of Americans with three or more chronic illnesses jumped from 7 percent to 13 percent in only 9 years after GMO foods were introduced. Autism, reproductive disorders, digestive problems, and other ailments have increased as well.

The American Academy of Environmental Medicine urges all doctors to prescribe non-GMO diets to patients, citing animal studies showing organ damage, gastrointestinal and immune system disorders, accelerated aging, and infertility. Although there have been fewer human studies on the risks of GMOs, they have proven GMOs leave material waste inside of our bodies, possibly attributing to long-term health issues.

As briefly mentioned earlier, doctors at the Sherbrooke University Hospital in Quebec found Bt toxin in genetically modified corn in the blood of pregnant women and their babies, as well as in women who weren't pregnant. The toxin was identified in 93 percent of 30 pregnant women, 80 percent of umbilical blood in their babies, and 67 percent of 39 women who weren't pregnant. The study has been accepted for publication in the peer-reviewed journal *Reproductive Toxicology*.

Due to these findings and their potential risks, at least 26 nations, including Switzerland, France, Australia, Austria, China, India, Germany, Russia, Japan, New Zealand, Greece, Mexico, Italy, Poland, and Mexico, have either total or partial bans on GMOs. About 60 other countries have significant restrictions on them. The United States, however, has no restriction on GMOs. In fact, they make up a vast majority of the produce on our shelves today.

How to Spot Non-GMO Food

If you live in one of the countries that has outlawed GMOs, you're lucky because to find non-GMO food, all you have to do is go to the market. If you live in the United States, however, it will be a little trickier. But with a little awareness, you can spot and avoid GMO food.

The best way to avoid GMOs in your food is to buy organic. Look for the Non-GMO Project Verified stamp on produce and other foods (and learn more at nongmoproject.org). Also, avoid any food that contains corn, soy, canola, or sugar beet, which are the most common GMO foods, unless they're specified non-GMO. Finally, purchase organic animal products to ensure they were not given GMO feed.

> **WISDOM OF THE AGES**
>
> Ayurveda recommends avoiding foods with toxins, including GMOs, rBGH, and pesticides. The best way to do that is to purchase organic foods. Organic foods also are more nutrient dense and better for your long-term health.

Foods Unstable for One's Doshic Constitution

The last reason you might develop a nutritional disorder is due to consuming the wrong food for your Doshic constitution. Many of us have imbalances we are unaware of. If you aren't consuming a diet for your unique needs, your body will spiral out of balance:

Vata: If you are a Vata type or have a Vata imbalance, consume Vata-pacifying foods like warm, cooked meals.

Pitta: If you are a Pitta type or have a Pitta imbalance, consume Pitta-pacifying foods with cooling, hydrating ingredients.

Kapha: If you are a Kapha type or have a Kapha imbalance, consume Kapha-pacifying foods like hot, spiced foods.

When you don't consume the right foods for your Doshic constitution, your digestion suffers. Digestion is the cornerstone of health, and if you aren't digesting your food properly, you'll begin experiencing imbalances unique to your Dosha:

Vata: Imbalances include bloating, gas, constipation, anxiety, and insomnia.

Pitta: Imbalances include heartburn, acidity, acne, increased body temperature, and anger.

Kapha: Imbalances include weight gain, lethargy, water retention, congestion, and allergies.

Be sure you consume the right foods for your unique Doshic constitution to avoid these imbalances.

The Least You Need to Know

- Ayurveda recognizes five types of nutritional disorders: quantitative dietary deficiency, qualitative dietary deficiency, quantitative and qualitative overnutrition, toxins in food, and foods unstable for one's Doshic constitution.

- Quantitative dietary deficiency is caused by not eating enough foods, and qualitative dietary deficiency is caused by not eating enough nutritional foods.

- Quantitative and qualitative overnutrition results from eating too much food, leading to obesity and diabetes.

- Toxins in our foods include GMOs, pesticides, and rBGH. Eating organic foods reduces exposure to these toxicities.

- Eating the wrong foods for your Doshic constitution can lead to a nutritional disorder. Your unique imbalances depend on your Dosha.

CHAPTER 14

The Seven Dhatus

"Head, shoulders, knees, and toes ...." That's how people learned to identify the various parts of the body at a young age. The childhood song definitely wouldn't be as catchy if it named the seven body parts in Ayurveda: "Plasma, bones, muscles, fat, nervous system, and reproductive system ...." Doesn't have quite the same ring to it, does it?

In this chapter, I discuss the seven dhatus, or bodily tissues where imbalances begin. Then I explain what these tissues are like in a healthy person versus in an unhealthy person so you can assess yourself.

In This Chapter

- The seven bodily tissues in Ayurveda
- Doshas and dhatus
- How our tissue health impacts how we feel
- Symptoms of dhatu imbalances

Meet the Dhatus

The *dhatus* are the seven tissue groups that make up your body. They are your plasma, bones, muscles, fat, nervous system, and reproductive system. Ayurveda identifies these areas to break down where disease manifests. You don't just get sick; rather, one area of your body becomes imbalanced, which affects the rest of it. By breaking down these tissues, you can pinpoint the location of your illness and treat that specific spot.

> **DEFINITION**
>
> The **dhatus** are the bodily tissue groups where disease manifests. You have seven in your body: plasma, bones, muscles, fat, nervous system, and reproductive system. It's important to learn about the dhatus so you know where your symptoms come from and how to treat them.

The Functions of the Dhatus

Each dhatu has a particular function:

- Your plasma provides your body with nutrition.

- Your red blood cells are in charge of circulating oxygen throughout your body and provide you with life.

- Your muscles provide strength and stability.

- Your fat, even if you dislike it, provides insulation and lubrication.

- Your bones hold your body together and protect your organs.

- Your bone marrow fills your bones and houses your nervous system.

- Your reproductive areas allow you to make and have babies.

You need all these layers to survive. These groups create the beautiful human body you live in.

How Ayurveda Sees Your Bodily Tissues

Ayurveda describes your dhatus in terms of qualities and relates them to the Doshas. Think about blood: it's red, hot, fiery, and full of life. Sounds like the Pitta Dosha, doesn't it? Thanks to a good understanding of the Doshas, you can better understand your bodily tissues.

Ayurveda further breaks down the psychological component of each tissue—remember, the mind and body are connected. The health of each body tissue connects to an aspect of your psyche. For example, your bones don't just provide your physical structure but also contribute to your mental stability. Building your *asthi dhatu*, or bone tissue, helps you stand up for yourself and become more confident in your beliefs.

AYURVEDIC ALERT

The state of your dhatu health is deeply related to your diet. You are a walking example of the foods you've consumed; your lunch will eventually become your organs, skin, and blood cells. If you consume unhealthy food, you won't have healthy body parts. You become whatever you put in your mouth, so be sure you eat nutritional food.

Dissecting the Dhatus

To give you a better understanding of the dhatus, let's look at what each dhatu is, what it connects to, its qualities, and the Doshas it relates to. After that, I explain what happens when the dhatu is healthy—or unhealthy—so you can see the implications in your everyday life.

There are two ways a dhatu can become imbalanced—either increased or decreased. I share the side effects of both so you can determine which you are experiencing and what Dosha it is connected to.

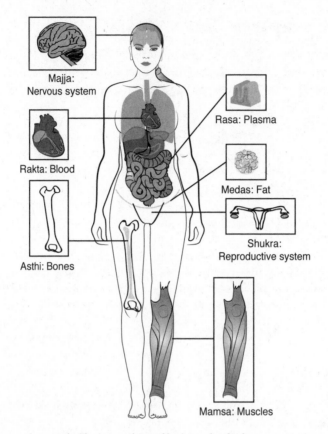

Majja:
Nervous system

Rasa: Plasma

Rakta: Blood

Medas: Fat

Asthi: Bones

Shukra:
Reproductive system

Mamsa: Muscles

Dhatus are the seven bodily tissues: plasma, blood, muscles, fat, bones, nervous system and reproductive system.

Rasa (Plasma)

The *rasa* dhatu is the juice of life. In fact, the word *rasa* means "juice" or "liquid." It refers to your plasma, which is the largest component of your blood, making up 55 percent of your overall blood content. When isolated, your plasma has a yellow color, which is also written in the Ayurvedic texts. Plasma carries water, along with salt and enzymes.

In Ayurveda, rasa is considered cold, heavy, moist, soft, stable, smooth, cloudy, gross, dull, and flowing, like the Kapha Dosha, comprised of water and earth. The purpose of rasa is to carry nutrients, hormones, and proteins to the parts of your body that need them. Your cells also deposit their waste in your plasma, and your plasma helps removes it from your body.

When rasa is healthy, you have good health, hormonal balance, physical beauty, mental clarity, and satisfaction. A person with high-quality rasa has soft, smooth, glowing skin; good energy;

and a creative mind. On the other hand, when rasa is unhealthy, you may experience breakouts, water retention, fear, or anxiety. Increased rasa causes congestion, colds, swelling, and a feeling of heaviness, which relates to the Kapha Dosha. Decreased rasa can cause constipation, dehydration, dizziness, dry skin, fatigue, irregular or loss of menstruation, and anxiety, all of which are related to the Vata Dosha. Decreased rasa caused by stress or excess spice in the diet is related to the Pitta Dosha.

Rasa depletion is caused by excess travel, overwork, stress, acidity, and/or too much spice in the diet. Excess rasa is caused by depression, weight-gain and/or inactivity.

> **WISDOM OF THE AGES**
>
> The health of your rasa is related to the health of your digestive fire. When the digestive fire is ideal, a healthy amount of rasa is produced with minimal amounts of waste. When the digestive fire is too weak, there is a great deal of waste, resulting in more rasa but poorer quality. When the digestive fire is too high, it burns through some of the rasa dhatu being created, causing a deficiency. A balanced digestive fire results in a balanced amount of rasa.

Rakta (Blood)

The *rakta* dhatu is the fire of the body. The word *rakta* means "reddened" or "impassioned" and refers to the blood in your body, specifically your red blood cells, as well as your tendons and bile. Rakta is the fire that invigorates your entire being.

In Ayurveda, rakta is considered hot, light, dry, hard, unstable, rough, flowing, clear, subtle, and sharp, like the Pitta Dosha, comprised of fire and water. The purpose of rakta is to energize and heat up your body. It also keeps your liver and spleen functioning properly so they can flush out toxins.

When rakta is healthy, you have a stable body temperature, strong blood circulation, robust endurance, and a passion for life. A person with high-quality rakta is motivated, ambitious, and active. On the other hand, when rakta is imbalanced, you experience cold body temperature, dull skin, and constipation.

Increased rakta causes excess sweat, increased body temperature, heavy menstruation, fever, tendonitis, and burnout, which relates to the Pitta Dosha. Decreased rakta causes bloating, gas, malabsorption, and a scanty period, which relates to the Vata Dosha.

Excess rakta is caused by stress, overexercise, and/or a spicy diet. Rakta depletion is caused by irregular eating habits, skipping meals, malabsorption, and/or malnutrition.

Mamsa (Muscles)

The *mamsa* dhatu is the muscular system of the body. The word *mamsa* means "meat" or "flesh." It refers to your muscles and also your ligaments, strength, vitality, and courage.

In Ayurveda, mamsa is considered hot, heavy, dry, hard, unstable, rough, dense, cloudy, gross, and sharp, a combination of the Pitta and Kapha Doshas. The purpose of mamsa is to provide a vessel in which you can live on this Earth. It is comprised of earth and fire energies, giving both substance and action.

When mamsa is especially developed, a person is born with strong muscularity and endurance. You also are self-confident and motivated in your actions. On the other hand, when mamsa is not adequate, you may be weak, prone to injury, inflexible, or lacking in self-confidence.

Increased mamsa causes a stiff body, tight muscles, and inflexible joints, which relate to the Kapha Dosha. Decreased mamsa causes low muscle mass, weak joints, tendency to toward injury, and hypermobility, which relate to the Vata Dosha.

Excess mamsa is caused by weight lifting, excess protein in the diet, and/or having a Pitta or Kapha Prakriti. Mamsa depletion is caused by inactivity, malnourishment, and/or having a Vata Prakriti.

Medas (Fat)

This probably is everyone's least-favorite dhatu—*medas,* or fat. Although some societies shame body fat, it's actually necessary for life. Fat is the way your body stores energy. It is necessary to protect your joints, balance your hormones, and keep you happy. However, too much can make you heavy and sluggish.

In Ayurveda, medas is considered cool, heavy, moist, hard, stable, and dense, like the Kapha Dosha. Those higher in Kapha naturally store more fat. However, this fat also lubricates the skin, which is why Kapha types have soft, smooth skin. Some fat is necessary for energy, but too much fat zaps it.

When medas is balanced, you have a healthy body weight and strong joints. When there's excess medas, you tend to be overweight, addicted to food, lonely, and lethargic.

Increased medas causes obesity, diabetes, joint pain, underactive thyroid, hypertension, excess thirst, breathlessness upon exertion, profuse sweating, and gallstones. Decreased medas causes dry skin, cracking and aching joints, cold body temperature, chills, loss of energy, irregular or lost period, infertility, emaciation, arthritis, osteoporosis, overactive thyroid, and enlarged spleen which relate to the Vata Dosha.

AYURVEDIC ALERT

Diminished medas, being underweight, is common today because of the Western perception of thin as beautiful. Many women purposely undereat to achieve this "ideal" body, which may not have enough fat for proper body function. If you are experiencing chills, lack of energy, loss of period, or joint pain, your medas may be out of balance, and it would be a good idea to consume a Vata-pacifying diet, with more warming, grounding foods and oils.

Excess medas is caused by overeating, lack of activity, excess carbohydrates and animal products in the diet, and/or a Kapha Prakriti. Diminished medas is caused by improper nutrition, overactivity, and/or a Vata Prakriti.

Asthi (Bones)

The *asthi* dhatu refers to your bone tissue. It is the densest dhatu in your body, made up 80 percent earth, 15 percent air, and 5 percent water. Ashti provides internal support, giving shape to your body and face. It protects your organs, including your brain, heart, and reproductive system.

In Ayurveda, ashti is considered cold, dense, hard, stable, and rough, similar mostly to the Kapha Dosha with a bit of Vata. Psychologically, asthi is the ability to stand up for yourself and be firm in your beliefs.

When asthi is healthy, you have a strong bone structure, teeth, nails, and hair. You are confident and assertive. On the other hand, when asthi is weak, you may have brittle nails, joint pain, hair loss, osteoporosis, arthritis, and scoliosis.

Increased asthi causes a bone fusion, bony protuberances/spurs, calcifications, hunchback, extra teeth, or excess hair growth, similar to the Kapha Dosha. Decreased asthi causes spontaneous fractures, arthritis, osteoporosis, brittle nails, hair loss, shortened height, and scoliosis, which relates to the Vata Dosha.

Excess asthi is caused by too much Kapha in the system and/or overconsumption of calcium. Diminished asthi is caused by excess Vata in the system, malnutrition, and/or lack of calcium and protein.

Majja (Nervous System)

The *majja* dhatu refers to your nervous system, although the word *majja* actually means "bone marrow" in Sanskrit. It's linked to the nervous system because the nerves exist within the vertebrae of the spinal cord. Majja is related to our sense of fulfillment.

There are two kinds of bone marrow. Red bone marrow is found in the spongy bones and produces red blood cells and hemoglobin, related to Pita. Yellow bone marrow is found in the medullary canal of long bones and stays in the canal to support the bone. Unresolved emotions can become stuck in the bone marrow, altering its properties; radiation and antibiotics can do the same. Psychologically, majja is the ability to communicate. Your brain shoots energy down your spinal cord, and that energy is prana. All your senses stem from your nervous system.

When majja is healthy, you are mentally stable, rich in energy, communicative, and your five senses (sight, hearing, smell, touch, and taste) are working properly. When majja is unhealthy, you may have anxiety, neurological disorders, hyperactivity, and hypoactivity.

Majja disorders can be caused by trauma; concussion; heavy metal toxicity; radiation exposure; alcohol, marijuana, or tobacco use; emotional stress; and poor diet.

Increased majja causes heaviness, sluggishness, thickening of skin, accumulation of fluid in ventricles of the brain, and tumors in the brain, related to the Kapha Dosha. Decreased majja causes anxiety, osteoporosis, anemia, multiple sclerosis, Parkinson's disease, epilepsy, attention-deficit/hyperactivity disorder (ADHD), lack of understanding, and poor communication, related to the Pitta Dosha.

> **WISDOM OF THE AGES**
>
> You can evaluate your majja by taking a look at your eyes. Eyes with dull grey eye whites and dry, crusty discharge indicate a Vata imbalance. Yellow-tinted eyes with a yellow discharge indicate a Pitta imbalance. Dull white eyes with an oily or mucous discharge indicate a Kapha imbalance.

Tears are a by-product of majja and how your nervous system discharges emotions. Allow yourself to cry and release any pent-up emotions you are holding on to in your nervous system.

Where tears fall from your eyes reveals what Dosha they are related to. Scanty tears that come from the outer corners of your eyes with a sweet taste are Kapha tears and often come from happiness or joy. Tears that fall from the center of your eyes and are hot and sour, often coming from anger, are related to Pitta. Tears that come from the inner corners of your eyes and come from frustration or intense grief are Vata tears.

Shukra (Reproductive Tissue)

Technically, the *shukra* dhatu relates to the male reproductive tissues and *artava* to female, but most modern Ayurvedic texts use shukra to refer to general reproduction. Shukra's great purpose is to produce life and continue the human species.

Shukra applies to sperm, testicle, and prostate health. It has a cool and active energy, predominantly Kapha but moved by Vata as well. Artava refers to menstruation and cervical, ovarian, and egg health. It's hot and passive in nature, relating more to Pitta.

When shukra/artava is healthy, you have a well-functioning reproductive system and creative instinct. When it's imbalanced, you may suffer from infertility, impotence, menstrual disorders, premature ejaculation, and low libido.

Increased shukra/artava causes sex addiction, premature ejaculation, excess semen flow, and multiple cystic ovaries. Decreased shukra causes lack of sex drive, pain during sex, impotence, and loss of menstruation.

Excess shukra/artava is caused by excess sexual activity and/or imbalanced hormones. Diminished shukra/artava is also caused by hormonal imbalance, as well as excess physical activity, low body weight, and/or increased Vata.

WISDOM OF THE AGES

Ayurveda states that the amount of sex one should have depends on the state of their shukra/artava, as well as their dharma, destiny. Those with a Kapha Prakriti can have sex the most often without depletion of their shukra/artava. Those with Pitta Prakritis can have moderate amounts of sex. Those with Vata Prakritis have lower levels of shukra/artava, thus risk getting depleted by having sex too often. Additionally, the more yoga and meditation one practices, the less sex they should be having, as these practices require a great deal of shukra/artava. This is why monks should remain celibate to build up their internal energy for their spiritual practice. Householders, on the other hand, should have sex to connect with their partner and reproduce, which is part of their dharma.

Dhatu	Related Body Part	Balanced	Increased Imbalance	Decreased Imbalance
Rasa	Plasma	Good health, hormonal balance, good energy, mental clarity, physical beauty	Congestion, colds, swelling, heaviness, acne, lethargy (Kapha)	Constipation, dehydration, dizziness, loss of menstruation, fatigue, anxiety (Vata)
Rakta	Red blood cells	Stable body temperature, strong blood circulation, motivation, endurance, passion	Excess sweating, increased body temperature, heavy periods, fever (Pitta)	Bloating, gas, malabsorption, scanty period (Vata)

continues

continued

Dhatu	Related Body Part	Balanced	Increased Imbalance	Decreased Imbalance
Mamsa	Muscles	Strong muscularity, ligaments, courage, vitality, self-confidence	Stiff and tight muscles, inflexible joints, heaviness (Kapha)	Weak joints, low muscle mass, tendency toward injury, hypermobility (Vata)
Medas	Fat	Healthy body weight, physical beauty, strong joints	Obesity, diabetes, hypertension, underactive thyroid, excess thirst, profuse sweating, breathlessness (Kapha)	Underweight, dry skin, cracking joints, cold body temperature, loss of energy, infertility, arthritis, osteoporosis, overactive thyroid, enlarged spleen (Vata)
Majja	Bone marrow (nervous system)	High energy, strong communication skills, great senses, mentally sound	Heaviness, lethargy, sluggishness (Kapha)	Anxiety, osteoporosis, anemia, multiple sclerosis, attention-deficit/hyperactivity disorder (ADHD), poor communication, epilepsy, Parkinson's disease (Vata)
Shukra (Artava)	Reproductive tissues	Well-functioning reproductive system, healthy sperm and egg health, creative instinct	Sex addiction, premature ejaculation, excess semen flow, multiple cystic ovaries (Pitta)	Lack of sex drive, pain during intercourse, impotence, loss of menstruation (Vata)

Healing the Dhatus

Now that you have identified which of your tissues may be out of balance, you are probably wondering what to do about it. This is where an Ayurvedic practitioner can help. Each of the Doshas can affect each of the dhatus, and only a trained professional will be able to evaluate your unique health. However, you can get an idea of what dietary and lifestyle changes to make by observing the Dosha it's connected to.

For example, if you have excess medas, fat, you can see that Kapha is at fault and follow a Kapha-reducing diet and lifestyle. If shukra is low and you've lost your sex drive or period, then Vata is off balance and you should follow a Vata-pacifying diet and lifestyle. Take a look at the symptoms of increased and decreased imbalance of each dhatu. When you find the one you relate to, notice what Dosha it connects to. Try following the dietary and lifestyle suggestions related to that Dosha for several months, and observe how your mind and body respond. Please consult with your doctor before making any changes.

Learning about the Doshas gives you the framework you need to treat unique areas of your body. Your physical body is deeply connected to your emotional. By understanding the dhatus, you can see how the health of your tissues contributes to high energy, creativity, and confidence.

Pay attention to the way you are feeling. If something feels off, it may be related to a deeper imbalance in your body.

The Least You Need to Know

- Each of your dhatus, or bodily tissues, plays an important physical and mental role in your well-being.
- The seven dhatus are plasma, bones, muscles, fat, nervous system, and reproductive system and the points where diseases begin.
- Dhatu imbalances come in two types: increased and decreased. The symptoms of each relate to the Doshas.
- You can treat your body by knowing what Dosha your dhatu imbalance is related to.

CHAPTER 15

Taste Is Everything

Many people believe they have to deprive themselves of flavor and taste to eat healthy, but Ayurveda states we must embrace them. Unlike modern diets that eliminate certain tastes, particularly sweet ones, the Ayurvedic diet calls for all six tastes in order to be nutritionally balanced.

Taste is much more than a delicious sensation in the mouth. The taste of a food tells you about its qualities, from the way it affects your body to how it impacts your mind. Sweet foods comfort while spicy pungent foods make you hot.

In this chapter, I explain what each of the six tastes are, the healthy and unhealthy foods you can find them in, and their effects on your mind and body.

In This Chapter

- How taste and nutrition are linked
- The six tastes you need every day
- The best and worst tastes for each Dosha
- Healing your body with tastes

How Taste Determines Nutrition

Ayurveda states that digestion begins the moment you put food in your mouth. Your mouth, including your tongue, lips, cheeks, roof of mouth, and even throat contains taste receptors, which signal to your body what enzymes are needed to break down your food. Just by tasting a food, your body knows what qualities the meal has. Genius, isn't it?

Most of us probably can only think of three or four tastes off the top of our heads, but Ayurveda classifies six tastes. Can you guess what they are? Think of all the tastes you are familiar with.

Most people immediately guess sweet, then maybe salty or sour. Savory is another common guess, but it's not actually a taste. Rather it's just a term that means "full of flavor." Likewise, spicy is not a taste but rather a flavor. Those who are more food savvy will guess bitter. In the Western world, people are taught that there are four tastes: sweet, sour, salty, and bitter. In fact, Plato and Aristotle both classified these four tastes, and modern scientists have agreed since. The Japanese have a fifth taste called *umami,* which is meaty and related to the amino acid L-glutamate.

In Ayurveda, the six tastes are called *rasas: madhura* (sweet), *amla* (sour), *lavana* (salty), *tikta* (bitter), *katu* (pungent), and *kashaya* (astringent).

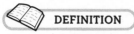

DEFINITION

The Sanskrit word **rasa** means "taste" as well as "juice," "flavor," "sap," "essence," "plasma," and "experience" because a taste is all those things. A rasa is your very first experience ingesting a substance, the flavor inside your mouth.

Madhura (Sweet)

The sweet taste, called *madhura,* is delicious, nurturing, and as you've surely experienced, highly addictive. Eating something sweet can feel like coming home, which is why sweets are so comforting and fulfilling. The sweet taste is high in Kapha Dosha, related to earth and water elements. In small amounts, sweet foods make you satiated and calm, but if you eat too much, you'll be left feeling heavy and uncomfortable.

Sweet foods are more than just sugar. Carbohydrates, including grains, fruit, bread, pasta, and starchy vegetables, are all considered sweet foods because they're still digested as sugar in the body. Milk and cheese are in the sweet category as well because they promote the same building qualities in your body.

Sweet foods include the following:

- Sweet fruits (bananas, mangoes, dates, figs, grapes, dried fruit)
- Starchy vegetables (sweet potatoes, squash, beets, carrots)
- Grains (rice, oats, couscous, barley)
- Wheat products (breads, pastas, pastries)
- Some dairy products (milks and cheeses)
- Sweeteners (honey, maple syrup, sugar)

Sweet foods build your seven bodily tissues, or dhatus, (remember those from Chapter 14?)—plasma, bones, muscles, fat, nervous system, and reproductive system. However, too much can result in excess of the least favorite bodily tissue, fat. The sweet taste is necessary for energy, organ production, endurance, and sustenance.

Children are naturally attracted to sweet foods because they're in the building Kapha stages of their lives, growing the bodies that will last them for their lifetime. Children gravitate toward candy, cake, and bread because their little bodies know they need something sweet to help them grow, even though simple carbs are not the best sources. Instead, they should consume naturally sweet foods like sweet potatoes and grains.

WISDOM OF THE AGES

Ever wondered how kids can live off sugar and still survive? It's because they are in the Kapha building stages of their lives and their bodies naturally crave sweet foods. Instead of feeding them candy, give them nature's candy: fruit.

Even though you are no longer in the building Kapha stage of your life, you need sweet foods in your diet, just in smaller amounts. The sweet taste is often vilified, but it actually has a lot of benefits. It increases moisture within your body, preventing dehydration and constipation. It soothes mucous membranes, balances hormones, relieves thirst, and increases saliva production. It's also necessary for beautiful skin and hair and even your voice.

Vatas need sweet foods the most to add structure to their frail bodies and balance their low hormonal levels. They may feel foggy-headed without enough healthy carbs in their diets. Vatas don't put on weight easily, requiring them to eat more sweet foods than the other Doshas to ensure they're getting the calories and energy they require. They need to pay particular attention to maintaining enough fat and muscle to protect their structures from injury and bone disease.

Pittas also benefit from sweet foods because they are highly active and their bodies require a great deal of energy. Sweet foods, particularly fruit, hydrate their bodies and cool them down. The sweet taste also is calming—something Pittas could really benefit from. They should avoid refined sugar and stick to more natural sources.

Kaphas need the least amount of sweet foods, even though they often love them the most. According to Ayurveda, like increases like and the sweet taste further imbalances already sweet Kaphas. Sweet foods unfortunately attribute to weight gain, lethargy, diabetes, and heart disease in excess. If you are overweight, constantly tired or congested, it is best to lower your intake of sweet foods, even fruit, and include more of the other tastes.

 AYURVEDIC ALERT

> Got a sweet tooth? You need more of the other tastes! Consuming more bitter, pungent, sour, astringent, and salty foods helps counterbalance the craving. For example, if you eat a sweet breakfast every day, try a savory one instead. It may reduce your cravings for the rest of the day.

Each taste affects your mind, as well as your body. The sweet taste, in moderation, is good for your soul. When you eat sweet foods, you feel happy. When you deny yourself of anything sweet for long periods of time, you might feel lifeless. This is why many people on highly restrictive diets are left feeling bitter—it may be all the bitter foods in their diet!

A little bit of sweet goes a long way, promoting compassion, love, and joy. Too much sweet food, however, can lead to qualities of laziness, greed, possessiveness, or attachment. That is why when you eat sweets every day, it's hard to let go—you literally have become attached to the substance!

To provide your body with its preferred source of energy, eat sweet foods every day from the right ingredients, like root vegetables, fresh fruit, and wholesome grains. That way, you don't crave refined sugar, which provides your body with the least beneficial source of sweetness.

Amla (Sour)

The sour taste, also called *amla*, increases your earth and fire elements—a bit of Kapha and a bit of Pitta. This makes it the best choice for Vatas, who could benefit from both. In fact, they often crave it. Sour foods increase stomach acid, improve digestion, and reduce flatulence, all things Vatas could really use. They also nourish your organs, blood, and other bodily tissues.

Sour foods include the following:

- Lemons
- Limes

- Grapefruit

- Apple cider vinegar

- Some dairy products, including yogurt, sour cream, kefir, and buttermilk

Think of a lemon. Imagine biting into its sour juiciness. Now notice your mouth. Have you begun salivating? Just thinking about sour foods is enough to increase your saliva production.

Digestion begins in the mouth, and the more lubricated your mouth, the more easily your body can digest your food. The acidic quality in sour foods helps break down foods, making them easier for Vatas to digest. Sour foods are energizing, invigorating, and often high in vitamin C with antioxidant qualities, particularly citrus fruits. They improve circulation and help your body extract minerals from your food, such as iron.

> **WISDOM OF THE AGES**
>
> Your body naturally craves the foods that are good for you, which is why Vatas crave sour foods. Sour foods moisten the mouth, stimulate saliva flow, increase stomach acid, enhance digestion, reduce flatulence, and clear dryness from the body.

Sour tastes bring out Pitta qualities. On the positive side, they increase alertness, sharpness, and attention span. However, excess sour can result in judgment, criticism, jealousy, and hatred.

Pittas should avoid eating sour foods if they have excess heat or itching in the body. Also avoid eating sour foods in hot, damp Pitta weather. Limes, pomegranates, and amalaki (an Indian fruit), are sour foods that are fine for Pittas because they have cooling and anti-inflammatory properties. Pittas should avoid fermented foods because they can lead to an acidic pH and heartburn. Too much sour food causes acne, hyperacidity, excess thirst, fever, diarrhea, eczema, itching, psoriasis, and ulcers in Pittas.

Kaphas can eat sour foods in small amounts. Apple cider vinegar is the best option for them because it promotes weight loss. A bit of lemon, lime, or grapefruit should be fine, too. Kaphas should avoid sour dairy products, which causes imbalances. A bit of sour foods may help reduce congestion, but excess will dry their mucous membranes and actually cause more congestion and dampness in the lungs. This is why Ayurveda is all about finding your own unique balance.

Lavana (Salty)

Salty is the third Ayurvedic taste and another favorite of many. Salty, or *lavana*, is comprised of water and fire energy, making it particularly high in Pitta energy as well as some Kapha. It's heat-inducing, oily, and heavy in nature. You require some salty tastes in your diet because it provides minerals, but too much can make you retain water.

Salty tastes include the following:

- Salt, of course (sea salt, rock salt, table salt)
- Seaweed
- Tamari
- Soy sauce
- Miso
- Celery (naturally high in sodium)

Salty foods are highly addictive because they enhance a food's flavor. However, too much salt overpowers every other flavor, making the food unpalatable. It also can lead to water retention, bloat, and dehydration.

The salty taste is energizing, promoting digestion, absorption, nutrient assimilation, and elimination, all qualities of Pitta. A bit of salt is also good for the body, encouraging muscle growth, preventing stiffness, and moistening the body. Salt encourages electrolyte balance and provides essential minerals. Salt soothes the nervous system and combats depression and a lack of creativity. It liquefies mucus and enhances skin glow.

However, the salt found in packaged foods, restaurant meals, frozen dinners, and canned soups is table salt, which is void of these great properties. Table salt contains high amounts of sodium without any nutritional value, leading to blood thickening, narrowed blood vessels, and high blood pressure (hypertension). This is why people must reduce their salt intake as they age.

> **WISDOM OF THE AGES**
>
> The salty taste isn't just in salt. Sea vegetables contain natural salts and minerals from the ocean. Fermented foods like tamari, soy sauce and miso are also high in salt content. Celery is a vegetable that is naturally sodium-rich.

Excess sodium also contributes to water retention, swelling, and puffiness, all qualities of Kapha. If you notice that your weight fluctuates greatly from the beginning to end of the day or your rings and jewelry are significantly tighter at night, try reducing your salt intake.

The reason you retain water with salt consumption is because salt actually dehydrates you. This causes your body to hold on to whatever water it can, making you heavier and puffier. You essentially turn into a walking water bottle!

The dehydration caused by excess salt is also a beauty disaster, attributing to wrinkles, baldness, gray hair, and dull skin. Excess salt wreaks havoc on your gastrointestinal tract, causing intestinal inflammation, ulcers, bleeding disorders, vomiting, and hyperacidity.

When it comes to salt, balance is key. It's important you consume high-quality salt in your diet to ensure you're getting the benefits. Try pink Himalayan sea salt, for example. Avoid table salt and packaged or frozen foods with excess sodium.

> **WISDOM OF THE AGES**
>
> A great way to be sure you get the salty taste without overdoing sodium is to eat foods naturally high in salt, such as sea vegetables, tamari, miso, and celery. These foods provide the minerals salt contains without the hypertension and swelling.

Katu (Pungent)

We don't use the word *pungent* as much in the English language, but we still often consume pungent foods without knowing it. Spicy foods, onion, garlic, and radish are all pungent.

The pungent taste, called *katu,* is heating, sharp, drying, and light, containing fire and air elements, a combination of Pitta and Vata. The taste is best for Kaphas because it contains the two elements they lack. A bit of pungent food can be good for Vatas because it's heating, but too much dries them out. Pittas should stay away from excess pungent foods because it overheats them.

Pungent foods include the following:

- Onions
- Garlic
- Chiles
- Radishes
- Mustard
- Black pepper, chili powder, cayenne
- Ginger

If you've ever bit into a chile pepper and started sweating, that's due to its pungency. Pungent foods promote sweating, detoxifying the system, and clearing out sinuses—another reason they're great for Kaphas.

Pungent foods stimulate the digestive fire, promoting digestion, assimilation, circulation, nutrient absorption, and detoxification. It's very common for cleanses to contain cayenne because of its metabolism-boosting qualities. Similarly, Ayurveda recommends spices for those seeking to lose weight, particularly Kaphas. Garlic is another great pungent ingredient to reduce candida yeast overgrowth and kill parasites.

The pungent taste brings out your Pitta qualities, both in a negative and positive way. If you are low in fire, pungent foods will make you sharper and more energized. However, if you have excess fire in your system, consuming pungent foods can make you irritable or angry. They also can cause physical Pitta imbalance symptoms such as hyperacidity, irritability, diarrhea, nausea, and ulcers. If you are high in Pitta energy already, it's best to consume small amounts of pungent foods, such as ginger or a bit of garlic in your cooking, and steer clear of super-spicy dishes.

Tikta (Bitter)

This is a taste that few people love but more of us need. Bitter, or *tikta*, is comprised of air and ether elements, high in Vata qualities. Bitter foods are detoxifying, anti-inflammatory, and cleansing. They also cause *lekhana*, a scraping of fat and toxins from your body.

Bitter tastes include the following:

- Leafy greens (kale, collard greens, dandelion greens)
- Brussels sprouts
- Zucchini
- Eggplant
- Bitter herbs (fenugreek, dill, neem)
- Turmeric
- Coffee
- Cacao

Bitter foods are extremely beneficial for digestion, which is why many people consume digestive bitters to aid in the breakdown of their meals. Bitter foods cleanse the liver and are antibiotic, antiparasitic, and antiseptic. Bitter bites also reduce intestinal gas and water retention, making them ideal for detox.

All three Doshas benefit from bitter foods, but Vatas should be careful not to overdo them because they may be too cleansing. Bitter vegetables are great for Vatas if they're paired with warming spices and oils, but extremely bitter herbs like neem and stimulants like coffee and cacao are not recommended for Vatas at all. Overconsumption of bitter tastes for already weak

Vatas can reduce bone marrow and make them at risk for osteoporosis. Excess bitter tastes also can reduce sperm production. In fact, Indian yogis often consume bitter neem to promote celibacy, both from sex and material possessions.

Pittas benefit from certain bitter foods, such as leafy greens and vegetables, but not others like coffee and cacao. Bitter foods stimulate the digestive fire but are still dry and light enough for Pittas with low digestive fire. Pittas are most susceptible to toxicities, which bitter ingredients can resolve. They also relieve burning sensations and nausea. Bitter foods reduce congestion and promote weight loss, making them a great option for Kaphas as well.

Kaphas benefit most from the bitter taste and are the only Dosha who can handle small amounts of coffee. Bitter vegetables and herbs are particularly medicinal for Kapha types because they alleviate thirst, reduce swelling, and promote weight loss. Bitter foods are energizing and detoxifying, promoting lekhana in heavy Kapha types.

> **WISDOM OF THE AGES**
>
> Has a fight left you feeling bitter? You may actually taste it in your mouth. You might taste a bitter residue in your mouth when you feel particularly lonely, isolated, or rejected. That's why you may crave sweets to help you get over it.

Kashaya (Astringent)

The last and least known of the six tastes is astringent. More than a taste, it's an effect on the tongue. If you've ever eaten something that left a dry taste in your mouth or caused you to pucker, that's astringent. The astringent taste, called *kashaya,* is used to describe dry, raw foods.

Astringent foods include the following:

- Raw broccoli, cauliflower, asparagus, brussels sprouts
- Artichokes
- Turnips
- Green beans
- Some legumes (chickpeas, yellow split peas)
- Pomegranates
- Cranberries
- Unripe bananas
- Turmeric (both bitter and astringent)

The astringent taste is cooling, drying, and heavy, comprised of air and earth elements, a bit of Vata and a bit of Kapha. Astringent foods are especially great for Pittas because they're so cooling and grounding. Astringent foods help bind the stool and combat diarrhea. They also are anti-inflammatory and heal ulcers and blood clots, exactly what Pittas need.

The astringent taste is healing for Kaphas in moderation because it helps scrape fat from the system (lekhana). Because astringent foods are drying, they can help combat water retention and swelling as well as tighten tissues. If you're a Kapha, just be sure you don't overdo it, because astringent foods are still cool and heavy, which are two characteristics Kaphas already have.

Vatas should minimize astringent foods because they are extremely cooling and airy, which may be difficult for Vatas' weak digestive systems to break down. Vatas do not do well with raw foods and have low blood pressure as it is, so excess astringent foods can make them weak and dizzy. However, small amounts of the astringent taste, especially turmeric and cooked astringent vegetables, are extremely healing. Include more astringent foods during the warm Pitta months, and reduce them in the colder Vata months.

Taste Chart

Taste	Action	Source	Dosha It Increases	Dosha It Decreases
Sweet	Building, calming, stabilizing, improves complexion	Grains, fruit, some dairy	Kapha	Vata, Pitta
Sour	Cleansing, aids digestion, balances cholesterol	Lemons, grapefruit, yogurt, fermented foods	Pitta, Kapha	Vata
Salty	Mineral rich, electrolytes, builds muscle strength	Sea salt, sea vegetables, celery	Pitta, Kapha	Vata
Pungent	Increases digestive fire and metabolism	Chili powder, cayenne, garlic, onions	Vata, Pitta	Kapha
Bitter	Detoxifying, scrapes fat, weight loss	Leafy greens, brussels sprouts, herbs, turmeric	Vata	Pitta, Kapha
Astringent	Scrapes fat, lowers blood pressure, anti-inflammatory	Raw vegetables, legumes, pomegranates, turmeric	Vata	Pitta, Kapha

What Should You Eat?

You should try to consume all six tastes every day to maintain balance, but you also should eat less of the tastes that imbalance your Doshic constitution.

If your Vata is out of balance, causing bloating, gas, and constipation, reduce foods that increase Vata (bitter, pungent, and astringent) and consume more foods that decrease it (sweet, sour, and salty).

If your Pitta is out of balance, causing heartburn, overheating, and high blood pressure, reduce foods that increase Pitta (sour, salty, and pungent) and increase foods that reduce it (sweet, bitter, and astringent).

If your Kapha is out of balance, causing weight gain, mucus, and lethargy, reduce foods that further increase your Kapha (sweet, sour, and salty) and increase foods that reduce it (bitter, pungent, and astringent).

The six tastes allow you to understand the nutritional qualities of your food without worrying about calories or nutrients. It's much easier to think about incorporating various tastes in your dishes than wondering whether you've gotten enough vitamin C or iodine in your meals. Tastes provide a delicious framework for healing your body that anyone can maintain.

The Least You Need to Know

- Ayurveda recognizes six tastes: madhura (sweet), amla (sour), lavana (salty), tikta (bitter), katu (pungent), and kashaya (astringent).
- Each taste has unique physical and mental effects on your body and your Dosha.
- To be healthy, you must include all six tastes in your diet but in varying amounts depending on what your Dosha needs.
- Vatas should favor sweet, sour, and salty foods and decrease pungent, bitter, and astringent tastes.
- Pittas should favor sweet, bitter, and astringent tastes and reduce sour, salty, and pungent foods.
- Kaphas should increase bitter, pungent, and astringent tastes and reduce sweet, sour, and salty ones.

CHAPTER 16

Breaking Down Digestion

When most of us think of digestion, we envision food going into our mouths, doing something in our bellies, and somehow ending up in the toilet. We aren't really sure what went on between those two very different stages but just know our guts have been up to something.

Digestion is a very tricky process, and sort of a miracle when you think about it. It takes your food and somehow turns it into your organs, brain, and energy. Pretty incredible if you ask me!

Ayurveda sees this miracle as the center of your entire well-being. It actually breaks down digestion into six unique stages, each lasting about 1-hour. Additionally, each stage is related to one of the six tastes mentioned in Chapter 15 and a Dosha. Everything in Ayurveda is so perfectly orchestrated, and the more you learn about it, the more you see the synchronicities.

In this chapter, I explain the six stages of digestion, the taste and Dosha each are related to, and what happens after you digest your food.

In This Chapter

- The six stages of digestion and the tastes they're related to
- Why snacking causes digestive disasters
- How fast each Dosha digests meals
- Clear colon = clear mind = clear life

The Six Stages of Digestion

The moment you put food in your mouth, the digestive process begins, and lasts approximately 6 hours, depending on what you ate. Ayurveda breaks down this entire process into six stages, each related to a taste. These stages are *madhura avastha paka* (sweet stage), *amla avastha paka* (sour stage), *lavana avastha paka* (salty stage), *katu avastha paka* (pungent stage), *tikta avastha paka* (bitter stage), and *kashaya avastha paka* (astringent stage).

These stages are related to the Doshas as well. The first two stages, sweet and sour, are related to Kapha because they are the heaviest. The next two stages, salty and pungent, are related to Pitta because they are when the stomach and intestines digest the food. The last two stages, bitter and astringent, are related to Vata because they are when the body becomes light again. Everyone go through all six stages, regardless of what their Dosha is.

> **WISDOM OF THE AGES**
>
> There are six stages of digestion, just as there are six tastes: sweet, sour, salty, pungent, bitter and astringent. In fact, the stages and tastes are related to one another.

Understanding the six stages of digestion helps you better understand your body. Oftentimes, you eat again before completing all six stages, causing digestive issues, toxic accumulation, and constipation. In this section, I break down each of the stages so you can get a glimpse of all the hard work your body has been up to and learn how to heal it if it gets a bit backed up.

Madhura Avastha Paka (Sweet Stage)

The first stage of digestion begins the moment food enters your mouth. According to Ayurveda, digestion starts as soon as your saliva and food meet. Your saliva begins the process of breaking down the food particles, which is why it's important to chew mindfully and thoroughly to give your saliva time to work.

In the first hour, you absorb your food's simple sugars and your blood sugar rises, which is why it's considered the sweet stage. The sweet stage is related to the Kapha Dosha because you often feel full and heavy after eating. Your earth and water elements increase, making you feel sedentary and sometimes a bit bloated after eating, especially after a big meal. However, if you eat the right amount, you'll just feel happily full and satisfied. That's why you feel so peaceful after a good meal—your Kapha is up!

> **WISDOM OF THE AGES**
>
> Modern science has shown that carbohydrate and fat digestion is initiated in the mouth. Amylase, the digestive enzyme that breaks down sugars, is produced by the salivary glands. Lipid (fat) digestion also begins in the mouth, called lingual lipase.

Amla Avastha Paka (Sour Stage)

The second stage of digestion is when hydrochloric acid in your stomach takes over to begin the digestive process. While carbohydrate and lipid digestion begins in the mouth, protein breakdown begins in the stomach. The stomach produces hydrochloric acid to denature the protein, destroy any bacteria/virus in the food and convert the digestive enzyme pepsinogen into its active version pepsin.

The second part of digestion is called the sour stage because your food becomes sour in your stomach. The stomach becomes extremely acidic to destroy any potential pathogens in your food, which is related to the Pitta Dosha. That's why those with a lot of Pitta have high levels of stomach acid and eating animal proteins boost it up.

At the same time, your stomach has to protect it's lining from the acid to prevent ulcers and other digestive issues, which is related to Kapha. For this reason, the salty stage is related to both Pitta and Kapha, as Pitta creates the acid and Kapha protects the stomach lining.

At this state of digestion, you may still feel a bit full and can sense the food in your stomach, although much less than you could during the first hour. This stage is comprised of both fire and earth energy; Pitta is fire, and Kapha is earth.

> **WISDOM OF THE AGES**
>
> If you eat excess acidic foods like meat without counterbalancing them with alkalizing foods, especially those high in protective Kapha energy like root vegetables, you may experience hyperacidity.

If you've ever broken out in hives or a rash after a meal, it was during the sour stage. The sour stage is when Pitta imbalances such as rashes, itching, and eczema take place.

Lavana Avastha Paka (Salty Stage)

The third stage of digestion is the salty stage. The food, now covered in stomach acid for about 30-60 minutes, enters the first part of your small intestine, called the duodenum. The duodenum prepares the partially digested food for absorption in the small intestine. The innermost layer, the mucosa, secretes alkaline mucus to neutralize the hydrochloric acid in the partially digested food. The food then mixes with bile from the liver and gallbladder, as well as pancreatic juices made by the pancreas to further breakdown the food. Peristalsis takes place, which are smooth waves of stomach contractions to push food through the duodenum, towards the jejunum. It takes about one hour for the food to travel the length of the duodenum.

This powerful stage of digestion is fully Pitta, comprised of fire and water elements. Your acidic food (fire) mixes with bile (fire) and pancreatic enzymes (water). The food is considered "salty" because of the meeting of the acidic food and alkaline digestive juices, like salt water.

The salty stage is extremely important because it's when you digest the carbohydrates, protein, and fats from your food. The pancreas secretes pancreatic juices that contain digestive enzymes: proteases, including trypsin and chymotrypsin, pancreatic lipase and amylase. Proteases digest proteins, while pancreatic lipase digests fats and amylase digests carbohydrates. Bicarbonate neutralizes the acid

 AYURVEDIC ALERT

It's in the salty stage of digestion that you must maintain a healthy electrolyte balance to prevent swelling, edema, or low kidney function, which are symptoms of insufficient or excess salt. Be weary of your sodium intake—you want to make sure you don't have too much or too little.

Katu Avastha Paka (Pungent Stage)

The fourth stage of digestion is the pungent stage and takes place in the jejunum, the next part of your small intestine. This stage is also related to the Pitta Dosha yet transitions into Vata, comprised of both fire and air energy. At this stage, your food is a yellow-brown color and filled with enzymes that have broken it down. This stage is hot, sharp, and subtle in quality.

If you have excess Pitta, the pungent stage is when you may experience overheating, hemorrhoids, skin rashes, or bleeding disorders due to excess fire. If you have excess Vata, you may experience gas and bloating due to excess air.

Tikta Avastha Paka (Bitter Stage)

The fifth stage of digestion is the bitter stage. The food has now traveled down to the final and longest portion of your small intestine, the ileum. It further digests with the help of air and ether, which govern movement and assimilation.

Air stimulates peristalsis, the involuntary constriction and relaxation of the intestinal muscles pushing the food down your intestines. Ether aids in the absorption of nutrients through the villi of the ileum wall.

During this stage, you often think you're hungry due to the light nature of the air and ether elements. However, it's important not to eat again until your body is done digesting your last meal so full absorption can occur.

> **AYURVEDIC ALERT**
>
> You may think you're hungry during the bitter stage of digestion when your stomach has started to lighten up. Do not make the mistake of eating until you have fully digested! If you put more food in your body before your last meal has been fully digested, you'll experience symptoms of toxic overload, including constipation, bloating, acne, and other digestive-related issues.

You may feel cold during this stage due to an increase of Vata energy.

Kashaya Avastha Paka (Astringent Stage)

The sixth and final stage of digestion is astringent. This stage is when you come full circle, your body has absorbed all the nutrients from your food, and the food has now turned into waste. This stage is comprised of both air and earth elements. Air causes peristalsis to push the food along your intestines, while earth creates the bulk of the stool.

In this stage, the food enters the cecum and the liquid foodstuff takes shape as it passes through the colon, preparing for elimination. Your stool not only contains food waste but other toxins from your body as well. After the food has been expelled, you begin to feel hungry again.

To make things more clear, the following table breaks down the stages of digestion and related information.

Six Stages of Digestion

Stage of Digestion	Taste Related To	Sanskrit Name	Elements	Dosha	Function
First	Sweet	Madhura	Water + earth	Kapha	Simple sugars are absorbed
Second	Sour	Amla	Fire + earth	Kapha + Pitta	Stomach acid is secreted

continues

Six Stages of Digestion (continued)

Stage of Digestion	Taste Related To	Sanskrit Name	Elements	Dosha	Function
Third	Salty	Lavana	Water + fire	Pitta	Food enters the top of the small intestine (duodenum); digestive enzymes are released
Fourth	Pungent	Katu	Air + fire	Pitta + Vata	Food enters the jejunum and continues to be digested
Fifth	Bitter	Tikta	Air + ether	Vata	Food enters the ileum; nutrients are absorbed
Sixth	Astringent	Kashaya	Air + earth	Vata + Kapha	Food enters the cecum and is formed into stool; appetite returns

Tips for Healthy Digestion

Now that you know the six stages of digestion and the actions that occur during each, you can appreciate how complex the digestive process really is. Your body is performing many tasks just to turn that salad into nutrients, and you can help it work more efficiently.

You might be doing things you think are healthy, like eating small meals throughout the day, that actually can be causing digestive problems. I explain how to avoid these potential disasters in this section. I also share how you can look out for a key indicator of your digestive health—one you probably are purposely overlooking.

Don't Snack Throughout the Day

Each of the six stages of digestion has a very important process that needs to be executed completely before moving on to the next. However, what happens if you keep eating throughout the day, like many Americans do? Your digestion will suffer, and your health will deteriorate.

Ayurveda is very against the snacking culture that exists today. It isn't good for you.

Nowadays, everywhere you go, people seem to be eating—while walking down the street, on public transportation, at their desk, at the gym, even while stuck in traffic. It seems like everywhere we go people have a smartphone in one hand and a snack in another. We have turned into a culture that revolves around food, yet with so little appreciation or knowledge about what we are putting into our mouths.

WISDOM OF THE AGES

People often eat for oral stimulation, rather than for physical hunger. When they are bored or in need of a break, they choose food rather than rest.

You've been taught to eat around the clock. In fact, the most health-conscious people are the ones eating the most often because the latest health fad calls for eating five to seven smaller meals a day to "keep your metabolism going." This couldn't be further from the truth. That actually hampers the digestive system and eventually leads to an even more sluggish metabolism, not to mention health imbalances.

Your body is designed to eat a meal, fully digest it, and then let you know when it's time to eat again. However, many people are too busy shoving food into their mouths to even know whether they actually are hungry or not. Eating has become a habit. But if you are constantly eating around the clock, you don't let your body perform the necessary six stages, which can cause toxic accumulation.

AYURVEDIC ALERT

By continually eating, you keep returning to stage one, the sweet Kapha stage of digestion. This suspends your body in a state of heaviness and promotes weight gain, lethargy, and water retention. If you don't wait the full length of the digestive process, you will never make it to the lightening bitter and astringent stages, when detoxification occurs.

The bitter stage is often when people eat again because they think they're hungry. What's really happening is your body is finally entering Vata stage so you feel lighter and emptier. It's easy to confuse that with hunger, especially if you're used to feeling full all the time. However, you have to let your body go through those final phases so it can detoxify the food waste in your system.

WISDOM OF THE AGES

Be sure to eat a meal substantial enough that you don't feel like you have to snack again 2 hours after. Each meal should contain all six tastes—sweet, sour, salty, pungent, bitter, and astringent. For example, a bowl of brown rice with vegetables sautéed in sesame oil, ginger, turmeric, and sea salt fulfills all six tastes, preventing you from craving more.

Schedule Your Digestion According to Your Dosha

We don't all digest food at the same rate. The rate of your digestion is affected by your Doshic constitution.

Pittas digest food faster and need timely meals or they become angry. They can eat every 4 hours and sometimes even get an acidic feeling in their stomach if it's left empty for too long. If Pittas eat before their digestive process has finished, they'll experience heartburn, ulcers, inflammation, and excess heat in the system. They don't do well with missing a meal because of their sharp appetites, which is why they should stick to their eating schedule.

Vatas have a variable digestive fire and should organize an eating routine so their bodies know when to expect food. They should wait 4 to 6 hours between meals. If Vatas eat before their digestive process has finished, they'll experience bloating, gas, and constipation due to excess buildup. Vatas, who tend to be grazers, should be sure they are eating meals substantial enough that they don't feel hungry in between. Protein and healthy fats, such as nuts and mung beans, are important to keep Vatas nourished and sustained.

Kaphas digest food the slowest and may be good with just two meals a day. They should wait a full 6 hours or until they truly are hungry before eating again. If Kaphas eat before their digestive process has finished, they'll experience lethargy, sluggish metabolism, water retention, and weight gain. Kaphas especially need to go through the two last stages of digestion, bitter and astringent. They cannot get away with snacking between meals because it will really add up for them. Their blood sugar levels are more sensitive than the other Doshas, attributing to weight gain. By constantly snacking, they'll remain in stage one, the sweet stage.

Kaphas should have a light breakfast and dinner and make lunch their biggest meal of the day. If they aren't hungry for breakfast or dinner, they can skip it. Their bodies store a lot of energy as body mass, so they are fine without a constant influx of calories and actually can benefit from fasting.

Knowing your Doshic constitution can help you determine how often you should be eating so you can allow your body to undergo the six stages. If you are somewhere in between two Doshas, follow the suggestions for that which is imbalanced:

> **WISDOM OF THE AGES**
>
> **Kapha imbalance:** If you are struggling to lose weight and have a sluggish metabolism, you are best eating less frequently, perhaps one or two meals a day.
>
> **Pitta imbalance:** If you have a sharp appetite and get an acidic feeling or sharp hunger pain when you don't eat, eat regularly every 4 hours.
>
> **Vata imbalance:** If you have a variable appetite, sometimes feeling hungry and other times not at all, set up a routine so your body knows when to expect food, every 4 to 6 hours.

Notice Your Bodily Cues

Notice your body's signals for hunger. Rather than eating just because you are tired, you're bored, or it's dinnertime, ask your body if it physically needs food.

Before you eat, ask yourself these questions: *When did I last eat? Is my stomach grumbling? Am I eating due to physical hunger or an emotional need? Have I waited until the last meal has fully digested? Am I able to sit down and mindfully enjoy this meal?*

If it's been 4 to 6 hours, you are physically hungry, and your answer to most of these questions is yes, then by all means eat and enjoy! However, if you just ate 2 hours ago and you aren't really hungry but rather just craving something sweet or salty, you'll inhibit your digestive process if you eat again. Wait until your body has fully digested before introducing more food in your system.

Subtract Before Adding

"Subtract before adding" means eliminating before you add more food to your system. Healthy bowels are key to a healthy body. Bowel movements result when your food has been fully digested, the nutrients have been absorbed, and the waste is eliminated.

Most people don't pay their stools much attention or even talk about them, but they're a daily indicator of their health. You should ideally be evacuating at least twice a day, with smooth, formed bowels. A healthy bowel movement has a smooth consistency and a light brown color, maintains its shape after being eliminated, floats, only has a mild odor, and does not stick to the toilet.

Don't be embarrassed if your stool is less than perfect. Most people's stools don't match these criteria. Do keep in mind it gives you an awareness of exactly what is going on in your body.

Your stool is like a stethoscope for your health. If your bowel movements are not up to par, there's something deeper going on inside of you that needs to be addressed. Instead of ignoring your bowels like they don't exist, pay attention to them and treat your body accordingly.

> **WISDOM OF THE AGES**
>
> Just by looking at your stool, you can see where your Doshic imbalances lay. Those with Vata imbalances have dry, hard, pelletlike stools, sort of like rabbit droppings. Those with Pitta imbalances have loose, watery stools that sometimes aren't fully formed. Those with Kapha imbalances have sticky, mucousy stools that often stick to the body or toilet.

Healthy elimination is crucial to clear toxins from your system. If you are not evacuating effectively, you become backed up, filled with the waste your body was supposed to discard. Over time, your entire digestive health will suffer, which leads to other illnesses from acne to anxiety. Ayurveda states that constipation is at the root of almost every disease.

The Least You Need to Know

- There are six stages of digestion, each associated with a taste.
- The first three stages are sweet, sour, and salty and when your body digests and begins breaking down food.
- The last three stages are pungent, bitter, and astringent and when you absorb the nutrients of your food and then push down the waste to be eliminated.
- Wait 4 to 6 hours between meals to eat again—don't snack—to allow your body time to undergo the whole digestive process.
- If you aren't eliminating smoothly and regularly, at least once in the morning, you likely are constipated.

CHAPTER 17

Ayurvedic Elemental Recipes

In Chapter 3, you read about the five elements that create the three Doshas: air, ether (space), water, fire, and earth. In this chapter, I discuss how you can determine what specific foods are related to each element. I then share 10 easy-to-make modernized Ayurvedic recipes related to each element so you can put all this wisdom to work.

Ayurveda is a kitchen science, and the real medicine is right on your plate. Let's get cooking!

In This Chapter

- The relationship among food, the elements, and the Doshas
- Fasting as a spiritual practice aid
- The elements you consume most versus what you need
- Easy, healthy recipes related to each element

Eat the Elements

The five elements exist all around us and combine to make up the three Doshas:

Vata: Air + ether

Pitta: Fire + water

Kapha: Earth + water

Notice how water exists in both Pitta and Kapha. How can that be when they are such different Doshas? Well, think about the qualities of water. Water can roll out of your hand, through the cracks between your fingers, practically weightless. Water also can demolish houses and create energy in dams. Water is both fluid and heavy, taking on different roles in the different Doshas. Water propels the transformation and energy creation in Pitta, while it grounds and hydrates the Kapha Dosha. This is why Pittas tend to sweat profusely and Kaphas tend to retain water.

To truly heal your body with food, you must understand the specific elements that make up each ingredient. For example, if you're a Kapha with a weak digestive system, you know you need more Pitta because that Dosha regulates digestion. However, if you consume more watery foods, you'll only become heavier because Kapha is already high in water. Instead, you need more fiery foods to stimulate your metabolism and boost your digestive system.

> **WISDOM OF THE AGES**
>
> Vata foods promote movement in the body because of their airy, etheric energy. Pitta foods promote transformation in the body because of their fire and water elemental powers. Kapha foods promote grounding and stability in the body because of the heaviness of their earth and water elements.

Understanding the elements gives you a deeper awareness of the foods you put in your body so you can achieve mind-body balance.

Let's look at the foods related to each of the elements and how they affect the Doshas.

Airy Foods

If someone has excess air in their body, what does that mean? Well, flatulence. It's literally air moving through your colon. You can think of the elements that factually.

Foods related to air are dry, rough, light, and fast-moving. Airy foods promote movement and lightness, making them ideal for weight loss. However, Vatas need to decrease airy ingredients because they already have so much air in their bodies. Excess airy foods cause bloating, constipation, and gas.

Pittas do best with airy foods because they lighten their sharp internal flames, which is what makes them so hot and bothered. The only exceptions of airy foods Pittas should minimize are nightshade vegetables, which include tomatoes, eggplants, and potatoes, because they cause hyperacidity in Pittas.

Kaphas do well with some airy foods because airy foods can lighten their heavy bodies and promote weight loss. Steamed cruciferous vegetables like kale, brussels sprouts, and cauliflower are great choices for Kapha types. However, Kaphas should stay away from cold and dry foods like popcorn, chips, and crackers because they're too cold for their already cool systems.

Each element has both healthy and unhealthy foods. Healthy airy foods include vegetables and beans. Raw and cruciferous vegetables are considered airy because they promote lightness in the body, but excess can cause bloat. Beans also are high in airy energy because as you know, they can make you gassy.

Unhealthy airy options include crackers and chips because they don't contain any nutritional value and are light and dry. Dried fruit is suitable for Pittas, although it is high in sugar. Popcorn is not traditionally Ayurvedic, but it's acceptable in small amounts if it's organic and non-GMO (genetically modified organism).

Airy foods include the following:

- Beans (black beans, chickpeas, etc.)
- Chips
- Crackers
- Cruciferous veggies (broccoli, cau-liflower, cabbage, brussels sprouts, kale)
- Dried fruit
- Popcorn
- Raw vegetables

Etheric Foods

The ether (space) energy is very similar to air, and people often get them confused. However, there is actually a difference between these two elements, which together create Vata.

Air relates to the air within your body, while ether relates to your relationship with what goes on *outside* your body. Air exists all around you, but ether is up above you. Air is within, while ether is without.

So how can you feel connected to ether? Think of it as a feeling of something greater than yourself. If you've ever drunk a really nutrient-rich juice and felt your cells vibrating with energy, that is ether energy. Similarly, if you've ever done a cleanse or fast and felt so good you were almost out of your body, that was ether energy you were feeling. Air refers to gassiness, movement, weight loss, and other internal factors. Ether relates to mental stimulation, consciousness, creativity, and your higher self.

Fasting is one of the main ways you can connect with ether energy. When you fast, you don't eat for a certain amount of time, whether it's several hours or even days. Some people even perform water fasts for weeks, although that's not recommended by Ayurveda. Ayurveda recommends keeping your fast to 1 day or doing a simple diet of just *kitchari*, mung beans and rice cooked in spices, for several days to get the benefits of fasting without the risks.

Many yogis and meditators fast regularly to connect to their higher selves. Taking a break from eating makes you less grounded in your body and more connected to universal consciousness. When you fast, you are no longer stuck thinking about when your next meal is going to come nor are you driven by hunger. This can really enhance your meditation practice. All the energy normally spent on digestion shoots upward, enhancing your third eye and crown chakras, which are in charge of intuition (more on chakras in Chapter 21). Many people report having clearer thoughts and more out-of-body experiences while fasting.

Fasting is recommended most for Kapha types, because they have extra energy on their bodies to help them stay nourished without food. In fact, Ayurveda recommends Kaphas do a 1-day fast once a week with just teas and juices during the day and a light soup at night. This gives Kapha bodies a break from digesting food and allows them to clear out any stored toxins. It also expands their creativity and brings stimulation to their sometimes dull minds.

Pittas also can fast on occasion—perhaps once a season. Pittas don't do as well with fasting because they need a constant influx of food. But once a season, a fast can help them detoxify and reboot their systems.

Vatas are not encouraged to fast. Because they are already so light, it can cause them to feel faint, weak, or malnourished. Interestingly, Vatas are most attracted to fasting because they love the feeling of being light and out of their body but they need it the least. Vatas require more grounding, not fasting. Kaphas are the least likely to want to fast, but they are the ones who need it most.

 AYURVEDIC ALERT

> Fasting can be a powerful practice to expand your meditation and help you connect with your higher self. Many fasters report feeling the subtle vibration of their own cells. Fasting takes your attention away from eating and turns it into your body. This is why fasting is so common in many spiritual practices across the world. Fasting is not recommended for Vata types, who are already light in energy. Kaphas are best suited for fasting, and Pittas can do it on occasion. Before undertaking a fast, please consult with your doctor. Try fasting for several hours first, then a day, and then expand your fast as you feel comfortable. To stay hydrated, continue drinking teas and/or juices.

Fasting is a means of connecting to ether energy, but foods also evoke similar qualities. Both positive and negative ingredients create that experience. Foods high in ether energy make you naturally feel uplifted, energized, and out of body. These include superfoods, green juices, sprouts, and coffee.

If you've ever felt you like wanted to take on the world after a cup of coffee or your cells were vibrating with nourishment after a refreshing green juice, that was ether energy. These beverages evoke etheric qualities because they literally give you a natural high. Green juice is recommended in the summer, especially when paired with ginger to make it more warming. Coffee is suitable in moderation for Kapha types but can cause anxiety in Vatas and irritability and acidity in Pittas.

Unhealthy ingredients that evoke ether energy include alcohol and drugs. Feeling drunk or high is an out-of-body experience yet not one that's conducive to your well-being.

Etheric foods and substances include the following:

- Fresh-pressed vegetable juices
- Spirulina, algae, and chlorella
- Maca, acai, and other superfoods
- Sprouts
- Coffee
- Alcohol
- Marijuana and other Drugs

Fiery Foods

Bring on the heat! Fiery foods increase Pitta energy and stimulate your agni, or digestive fire. These foods make you sharp and motivated, but excess leaves you feeling hot and bothered. Fiery foods stimulate your metabolism and enhance your digestion, making them especially great choices for Vatas and Kaphas, who lack in fire energy. However, Pittas need to be careful not to overdo the fiery foods, even though they are attracted to them, because excess can make them overheated, acidic, and impatient.

Fiery foods are best to have in the winter, when you're low in internal heat. Excess fiery foods in the summer can make you overheated and irritable.

Healthy fiery foods include spices, hot peppers (chile, black, cayenne), onions, garlic, and even sour fruits, which are all high in Pitta energy. Coffee is high in fire energy as well because it makes you literally hot and stimulates the fire within. It's least recommended for Pitta types and most for Kaphas. The best fiery ingredients are spices like ginger, cloves, cinnamon, and cumin, which can be added to your meals to enhance your digestive fire.

Unhealthy fiery substances include alcohol and tobacco. Notice how alcohol is also both high in ether and fire energies, like coffee. That is because alcohol is a stimulant that makes you feel both out of body but also aggravated and overheated within your body. Ayurveda does not recommend alcohol in any capacity because it is so dehydrating and acidic. Similarly, tobacco is not recommended.

Fiery foods and substances include the following:

- Ginger, cloves, cinnamon, cumin, asafetida, and other warming spices
- Black, cayenne, chile and other hot peppers
- Sour fruits (lemons, grapefruit, tamarind, pineapple, and cranberries)

- Pungent onions and garlic
- Coffee
- Alcohol
- Tobacco

Watery Foods

Water is the element you contain the most of. Around 65 percent of your body is made of this liquid element. Watery ingredients hydrate your body, which make them a great choice for dehydrated Vatas and overheated Pittas. Too much, however, can make Kaphas heavy and puffy because they easily retain water.

Watery ingredients are best during the hot summer Pitta months, when you could benefit from extra hydration in your diet. Juicy fruits and vegetables are the best sources of water in your diet. Salt is related to the water element because it causes your body to retain hydration. Dairy products are related to water as well because they are cool and damp, like water.

Vatas should consume more watery ingredients in summer and less in winter because they can be overly cooling. Pittas should favor juicy fruits and vegetables but minimize dairy and salt. Kaphas should avoid excess watery ingredients because they cause them to retain water, leaving them bloated and puffy. Kaphas especially must stay away from dairy products, which cause mucus and inflammation in their systems.

Watery foods include the following:

- Juicy fruits (watermelon, papayas, oranges, cantaloupe)
- Avocados
- Coconut water and oil

- Juicy vegetables (cucumbers, zucchini, tomatoes)
- Dairy products
- Salt

Earthy Foods

Foods high in earth energy are extremely grounding and nourishing. They often are grown under the ground and carry those rooted properties with them. Earthy foods give your body stability and structure, making them a particularly great choice for weak, airy Vata types who lack in grounding. Any food that is dense and heavy is considered an earthy food. They provide energy, endurance, and strength, high in Kapha qualities.

Earthy ingredients are great for Pittas, too, because they calm them and ease their sharp digestive fire. The only earthy food Pittas should avoid is nuts because they can cause oiliness and breakouts.

Kaphas are naturally high in earth energy and don't need as much as the other Doshas. Kaphas can have earthy vegetables, beans, mushrooms, seeds, and grains that are also high in air or fire energy because they will be lighter to digest. However, they should steer clear of excess nuts and coconut meat, which are very calorically dense and can add up.

Earthy foods include the following:

- Root vegetables (yams, squash, pumpkins, beets, turnips, parsnips, carrots)
- Most nuts and seeds
- Mushrooms
- Beans
- Most grains
- Coconut meat

How's Your Diet?

Now that you know the ingredients related to each element, let's look at your diet.

Which element is most prevalent in your diet? Which do you least consume? Which element could you use more of? How can you incorporate more of that element's foods in your meals?

For an easy way to incorporate the necessary element's foods in your menu, keep reading. In the following sections, I offer 10 recipes you can choose from related to each element.

I offer more element-related recipes on my website eatfeelfresh.com. You can search through recipes by ingredient, Dosha, or element to build your menu of healing recipes.

 WISDOM OF THE AGES

The elements have particular functions in your body. Air, ether, and fire energies are light and move upward, making you feel uplifted and energized. Earth and water energies move downward, making you feel heavy and rooted. That is why Kaphas often feel lethargic and slow while Vatas and Pittas feel more energized. You must balance your Dosha with the opposite qualities in your diet. Vatas and Pittas could benefit from more grounding in their diet, while Kaphas need more uplifting.

Recipes for Each Element

At this point, you know about the elements, foods related to each, and what you need more and less of. Yet you might be wondering how to make that happen, especially if you have little to no experience in the kitchen. Don't worry. I've got you covered.

In this section, I give you two recipes related to each element. I also share options on ways to customize the recipes for each Dosha so you can enjoy them regardless of your constitution. Remember, you need all the elements in your diet, just in various amounts.

Vatas should favor more fiery and earthy recipes but can consume airy, etheric, and watery recipes as long as they make them warming. Pittas should favor earthy, watery, airy, and etheric recipes but can consume fiery recipes as long as they aren't spicy and don't have too much garlic or nightshades. Kaphas should favor airy, etheric, and fiery recipes but can consume watery and earthy dishes as long as they don't make them too grounded and heavy.

Ready to get cooking?

Airy Recipes

Airy recipes evoke lightness in the body. Cruciferous vegetables are one of the best ways you can increase the air element while staying balanced. I've included two cooked cruciferous vegetables, one smooth and one crunchy, that can work for all three Doshas with slight modifications.

Cauliflower Mashed "Potatoes"

Mashed potatoes are comfort food. You can lighten them up by replacing the potatoes with cauliflower and reduce the calories and carbs. This recipe works for all three Doshas because it is cooked and mashed, easy for Vatas to digest and light enough for Pittas and Kaphas. Pittas should reduce the garlic, and Kaphas should reduce the oil.

1 large head cauliflower, florets roughly chopped	$1/2$ cup unsweetened almond milk (not vanilla flavored)
1 or 2 TB. olive oil	$1/2$ tsp. sea salt
1 or 2 cloves garlic	$1/4$ tsp. freshly ground black pepper
1 large leek	2 TB. fresh chopped chives (optional)
1 TB. ghee or vegan butter	1 tsp. fresh thyme (optional)

1. In a large pan over medium-high heat, boil cauliflower in water to cover for 7 to 10 minutes or until soft. Remove from heat, drain, and set aside cauliflower to cool.

2. In a medium skillet over medium heat, heat olive oil. Add garlic and leek, and sauté for 3 or 4 minutes or until leek is tender. Remove from heat.

3. In a food processor fitted with an S-blade, or in a blender, blend cauliflower, garlic, leak, ghee, almond milk, sea salt, black pepper, chives (if using), and thyme (if using) until creamy and smooth.

4. Serve warm.

An alternate way to make this recipe is to steam the cauliflower with the garlic and leek until soft for about 20-30 minutes, then use an immersion blender to combine it with the ghee, almond milk, and spices.

Brussels Sprout Chips

Chips are crunchy, satisfying, and addictive. This brussels sprout version allows you to eat a handful of chips while still getting your daily veggie intake. Best of all, they only take 10 minutes to bake. Vatas with extremely weak digestive systems may have bloating with brussels sprouts.

10 brussels sprouts

1 TB. extra-virgin olive oil

$1/4$ tsp. sea salt

$1/2$ TB. dried oregano, cilantro or basil (optional)

$1/2$ TB. dried turmeric (optional)

1. Preheat the oven to 350°F. Line a baking sheet with parchment paper.

2. Wash brussels sprouts and dry in a salad spinner to make sure they're completely dry. Place on a cutting board and using a paring knife, chop off bottom tip of each sprout. This will cause outer leaves to begin to fall off. Continue trimming a little more off the bottom so leaves all fall off.

3. Place brussels sprout leaves in a large bowl with olive oil, sea salt, herbs or turmeric (if using), and toss to coat. Spread brussels sprout leaves in a single layer on the prepared baking sheet.

4. Roast for about 10 minutes or until chips are lightly browned and crisp. For best results, turn them after 5 minutes. They should look crunchy and almost burnt, but not quite. Allow to cool, and enjoy.

WISDOM OF THE AGES

It's easy to overeat regular potato or corn chips because they feel so light in our hands and mouths, causing us to underestimate the caloric load—especially dangerous when they're deep-fried in hydrogenated oil. You can enjoy this baked brussels sprout version instead without any guilt.

Etheric Recipes

Ether-inducing foods promote vibrancy and higher consciousness They're the type of foods that light you from within and give you out-of-body energy.

One of my favorite etheric ingredients is a blue-green microalgae called spirulina that dates back 3.5 billion years. Packed with protein; iron; docosahexaenoic acid (DHA); vitamins B, C, A, K, and E; calcium; potassium; magnesium; beta-carotene; and other vitamins and minerals, spirulina is one of the most nutrient-dense foods on the planet. It's particularly great for vegans because it's about 60 percent pure protein and very high in iron and vitamin B. Just be careful not to cook spirulina because its living enzymes will die. Spirulina is great for all three Doshas and can be added to juices and raw meals to amp up the nutritional benefits.

Spirulina Green Juice

One of the best ways to consume spirulina is in a green juice. Pittas do best with green juices because they're so alkalizing. Green juices can be too cooling for Vatas and Kaphas with weak digestive fires, so they should only have them if they don't experience negative side effects. Adding ginger is a great way to crank up the warming factor of green juices. Green juices are best consumed in the hot, Pitta months because they are so cooling. Kaphas can omit the apple to make it totally sugar free.

1 large organic English cucumber

1 head kale, roughly chopped

1 ($^1/_2$-in.) piece unpeeled ginger

1 large organic lemon or lime, peeled if not organic or not peeled if organic as the skin is highly nutritious

1 cored green apple, with skin

1 tsp. spirulina powder

1. In a juicer (or a blender if you don't have a juicer), juice English cucumber, kale, ginger, lemon, apple, and spirulina powder.

2. Drink within 15 minutes of juicing for maximum benefit.

WISDOM OF THE AGES

Although not traditionally Ayurvedic, green juices can ensure you get your daily greens with just one cup.

Detoxifying Spirulina Dressing

Spirulina is a great additive to dressings and sauces. Salads are traditionally not Ayurvedic but can work for those with strong digestive fires or during the hot, summer months. Kaphas can reduce the oil, and Pittas can omit the garlic powder.

1 or 2 TB. extra-virgin olive oil

1 TB. apple cider vinegar

1 tsp. spirulina powder

Juice of 1 large organic lemon

1 tsp. garlic powder

1. In a small bowl, whisk together extra-virgin olive oil, apple cider vinegar, spirulina, lemon juice, and garlic powder.

2. Use to dress a salad, or pour over roasted, steamed, or raw vegetables, depending on your Doshic needs.

Spirulina offers a slightly parmesan-cheese-like taste to salads and makes a great replacement for traditional dairy cheese.

Fiery Recipes

Fiery recipes are perfect for those cold winter days when you feel chilled to the bone. They stoke your digestive fire and provide warmth, circulation, and satiety. Spices are one of the best sources of the fire element because they work both as food and medicine. Each spice contains unique benefits, from bloat reduction to joint pain relief, making them the most delicious prescription you'll ever have.

Spices can be used in foods as well as beverages. Teas, curries, stir-fries, soups, and bakes all can benefit from a sprinkle of spice. Pittas should be careful not to overdo the especially fiery spices, like cayenne and jalapeño, because they can overfeed their fire.

Spicy Digestion-Enhancing Veggie Stir-Fry

This is one of my favorite stir-fry recipes because it's extra stimulating for the digestive fire. Pittas should choose coconut oil and omit the garlic, jalapeño, and mustard seeds. Vatas and Kaphas should choose sesame oil and can feel free to crank up the spice amounts.

1 TB. mustard seeds

2 TB. sesame or coconut oil

1 medium yellow onion, chopped

1 clove garlic, minced

1 (1-in.) piece ginger, peeled and grated (1 TB.)

$^1/_2$ jalapeño, ribs and seeds removed and chopped

2 cups chopped asparagus, carrots, brussels sprouts, bell peppers, cabbage, butternut squash, or your choice vegetables

1. Heat a large skillet over medium heat. Add mustard seeds, and dry toast for 3 minutes or until you hear a popping sound.

2. Add 1 tablespoon sesame or coconut oil, onion, garlic, and ginger to the skillet, and sauté for 3 minutes or until onion is golden brown.

3. Add jalapeño, chopped vegetables, and remaining 1 tablespoon oil, and sauté for 5 minutes or until vegetables are tender.

4. Serve warm alongside your favorite grain.

WISDOM OF THE AGES

It's easy to get your spices in with a quick stir-fry filled with your favorite veggies. The best part about a stir-fry is you can customize the ingredients to use what's local, seasonal, and required for your Doshic needs.

To give this dish a more Asian feel, add tamari or coconut aminos, which are low-sodium replacements for soy sauce, rice vinegar and scallions.

Warming Spiced Masala Chai

Chai is a classic Ayurvedic recipe comprised of aromatic ginger, cloves, star anise, peppercorns, and cardamom steeped in black tea. *Chai* is the word for "tea" in Hindi, and *masala* means "spiced," so *masala chai* literally means "spiced tea." Unlike other teas brewed in water, the spices of chai are brewed in milk, giving the beverage its fragrant qualities. In this sugar-free, plant-based version, I've replaced the dairy milk and sugar with almond milk and monk fruit sweetener. You could use stevia, maple syrup, or honey if you like. Pittas should omit the peppercorns.

2 bags black tea

1 whole star anise pod

2 tsp. ground cinnamon or 1 cinnamon stick

4 dried cardamom pods

1 (1-in.) piece ginger, peeled and grated (1 TB.)

1 tsp. whole black peppercorns (optional)

2 cups almond milk

1 TB. monk fruit sweetener or to taste

1. In a small saucepan over medium heat, warm black tea, star anise, cinnamon, cardamom pods, ginger, peppercorns (if using), and almond milk for 7-10 minutes. Remove from heat when mixture begins to bubble but before it boils.

2. Strain mixture into a cup, add monk fruit sweetener, and enjoy. (You also can leave the spices in your cup, which is what I do.)

WISDOM OF THE AGES

Historically, Indians viewed tea as an herbal medicine rather than a recreational beverage. The recipes came directly from Ayurvedic medical texts, and indicated tea was meant to heal, not entertain. During their rule in the 1830s, the British began cultivating tea plantations in India, and in the early 1900s, Britain set up the Indian Tea Association and encouraged Indians to begin drinking tea. Today, Indians enjoy several cups of warm chai a day, savoring it as a much needed break.

Watery Recipes

You know it's essential that you drink enough water every day, but how much attention do you pay to how much water you *eat?* Juicy fruits and vegetables are a great way to ensure you stay hydrated without taking a sip. They are naturally high in water content, making them especially hydrating as well as low in calories. Watery ingredients cool the body and prevent constipation, which is caused by dryness.

The ideal time to consume watery foods is in the summer, which happens to be when they grow. Pittas should favor juicy fruits like papayas and watermelons and vegetables like cucumbers and zucchini. Stay away from nightshades like tomatoes and eggplants. Vatas do well with most watery ingredients but shouldn't have excess in the winter because it may be too cold for them. That's why I added ginger to the following recipe. Kaphas should add ginger to heat up their meals but shouldn't have too many juicy ingredients because it can make them to retain more water.

Refreshing Coconut, Ginger, Lime, Papaya "Lassi"

Chances are you've seen or tried a mango lassi at an Indian restaurant. This Indian smoothie, made with mango, a fermented yogurt beverage, and a sweetener, isn't actually Ayurvedic because it doesn't follow food-combining rules. I've upgraded the recipe to make it lower in sugar, easier to digest, plant based, and agreeable for all three Doshas. I've replaced mango with papaya because papaya is lower in sugar and also great for digestion. I've replaced the lassi with coconut milk, which is plant based and doesn't contain mucus-causing dairy. I've added ginger and cardamom to make it more warming to digest, as well as lime to include the detoxifying sour taste. These ingredients balance out the smoothie so it works with all three Doshas.

1 cup ripe papaya, cubed

1 ($^1/_2$-in.) piece ginger, peeled and minced ($^1/_2$ TB.)

1 tsp. cardamom

Juice of 1 small, juicy lime

1 cup coconut milk

1. In a blender, combine papaya, ginger, cardamom, lime juice, and coconut milk until smooth.

2. Enjoy immediately.

WISDOM OF THE AGES

Ayurveda advises against combining fruit with dairy. Fruit should always be consumed alone on an empty stomach, without any other ingredients, according to Ayurvedic texts. And dairy products are heavy and dense and should be eaten separately because they take longer to digest. You don't have to worry about that with this refreshingly tart yet sweet recipe!

Cooling Cucumber Zucchini Soup

This is a perfect go-to summer recipe when you're looking for an easy dinner with little preparation work. The soup contains moisturizing avocado, hydrating zucchini, cooling cucumber, sweet onion, and cleansing coriander, all of which detoxify and refresh your body. Best of all, no cooking is required! Pittas should remove the hot green chile.

3 medium zucchini, chopped

$^1/_2$ large organic seedless cucumber, chopped

$^1/_2$ medium sweet onion, chopped

1 medium ripe avocado, peeled and pitted

$^1/_4$ cup water

1 tsp. chopped fresh hot green Hatch chile

1 tsp. sea salt

1 tsp. ground coriander

1. In a blender, combine zucchini, cucumber, sweet onion, avocado, hot green chile, sea salt, and coriander until smooth.

2. Enjoy immediately.

Earthy Recipes

Earthy recipes provide the grounding qualities that really bring you back to your nature. They're perfect for when you're feeling stressed out or too in your head and need to settle your body and your mind. They also help soothe digestive issues, including bloating or gas.

Root vegetables are one of the best earth-containing ingredients you can consume because they are literally grown in the soil. You take on the qualities of the food you eat, and earthy ingredients are rich with natural qualities and deeply rooted. Vatas and Pittas benefit most from earthy tastes, but Kaphas can consume them as well if they add heating spices like ginger, garlic, and cumin to aid their digestive fire.

Spiced Butternut Squash Soup

Butternut squash is an earthy, fall classic—warming, grounding, sweet, and straight from the soil. When paired with warming spices, it's especially nourishing. This recipe works for all three Doshas because the coconut milk lightens it for Pittas and the spices make it more stimulating for Kaphas. Pittas should choose coconut oil and omit the garlic. Vatas and Pittas should choose sesame oil and can add more spices as they like.

1 TB. coconut or sesame oil	1$^1/_2$ cups coconut milk
2 cloves garlic, minced	2 cups low-sodium vegetable broth
$^1/_2$ medium yellow onion, chopped	1 ($^1/_2$-in.) piece ginger, peeled and grated ($^1/_2$ TB.)
1 small butternut squash, chopped, peeled, and seeded	2 TB. maple syrup or honey (optional)
2 TB. curry powder	Pinch sea salt
1 tsp. turmeric	Pinch black pepper
$^1/_2$ TB. ground cinnamon	

1. In a large pot over medium heat, heat coconut or sesame oil. Add garlic and yellow onion, and sauté for 3 minutes or until onion is golden brown.

2. Add butternut squash, curry powder, turmeric, and cinnamon. Cover and cook, stirring occasionally, for 10 minutes.

3. Add coconut milk, vegetable broth, ginger, maple syrup (if using), sea salt, and black pepper.

4. Bring to a boil, reduce heat to low, cover, and simmer for 15 minutes or until butternut squash is cooked through.

5. Remove from heat, and allow to cool.

6. Blend soup until creamy and smooth using an immersion blender or by transferring to a blender in batches. (If transferring to a blender, be sure soup is well cooled to prevent an explosion from the blender.)

7. Enjoy immediately, or warm again before serving.

Ayurvedic Beetroot Hummus

Hummus is an easy source of protein. You can pair it with any type of veggie or grain or serve it as a salad dressing. Beetroot is a great way of adding more grounding elements to classic chickpea hummus because beets are root vegetables. Beets also provide a bit of sweetness, making them especially nourishing for Vata and Pitta Doshas. Consuming beets can prevent Kaphas from having sweet cravings because they naturally satisfy their sweet tooth. Because hummus is cold, I added warming spices to this recipe to make it easier to digest for sensitive Vatas and Kaphas. Pittas should omit the garlic.

1 small beetroot

1 TB. sesame or olive oil

2 cups chickpeas, soaked in 4 cups water overnight or at least 5 hours

2 TB. tahini

2 large cloves garlic, minced

1 tsp. cumin

Juice of $^1/_2$ lemon

2 tsp. sea salt

Healthy pinch black pepper

4 cups and 1 TB. water

1 or 2 TB. extra-virgin olive oil (less for Kaphas)

1. Rinse chickpeas with water and place in a large pot with 4 cups water and 1 tsp. sea salt. Bring to boil. Cover the pot and simmer until chickpeas are soft all the way through, which takes between 30-45 minutes, depending on how long you soaked the chickpeas for. Drain the excess water.

2. Preheat the oven to 375°F.

3. Remove beetroot stem and roots, and wash clean. Wrap beetroot in aluminum foil with 1 TB. sesame oil, and roast for 1 hour. Allow to cool and peel.

4. In a food processor fitted with an S-blade, or in a blender, blend beetroot, chickpeas, tahini, garlic, cumin, lemon juice, sea salt, and black pepper until smooth. If hummus is too dry, add water and blend again.

5. Transfer hummus to a serving bowl, drizzle olive oil over top, and serve with veggies.

The Least You Need to Know

- You can restore balance to your body through your diet by eating the elements you are lacking.
- Raw and cruciferous vegetables are examples of airy foods.
- Juices and spirulina are examples of etheric foods.
- Ginger and chile peppers are examples of fiery foods.
- Papaya and cucumbers are examples of watery foods.
- Root vegetables and nuts are examples of earthy foods.

CHAPTER 18

Common Ayurvedic Diet Questions

I'm sure you've had questions as you've been reading this book. I know how frustrating it can be to have unanswered questions, especially on such a potentially confusing subject. So in this chapter, I want to go over some queries you might have about leading an Ayurvedic lifestyle.

In the following sections, I explain exactly what ingredients and supplies you need, teach you how to cook for a family of different Doshas, go over ways to overcome cooking blocks, share tips on timing your meals, and much more.

By the end of this chapter, you'll be an Ayurvedic-cooking pro, ready to heal your friends and family with medicinal meals.

In This Chapter

- How you can eat Ayurvedically, even if you don't know how to cook or don't have the time or money

- The staples you need in your Ayurvedic kitchen and which you should buy organically

- What to order at a restaurant in-line with Ayurvedic guidelines

- My simple 10-week plan to becoming an Ayurveda pro by only changing one habit a week

Questions About Ayurvedic Cooking

Ayurvedic cooking is one of the most intuitive methods of preparing food possible. It doesn't have strict rules like French or other cuisines. Rather, you cook what's local and seasonal, and pair it with a variety of aromatic spices and herbs.

Let's go through some questions you may have when it comes to Ayurvedic cooking so you feel comfortable in the kitchen.

What If You Don't Know How to Cook?

One of the best parts about Ayurvedic recipes is their simplicity. You don't need any culinary experience to whip up an Ayurvedic meal. All it takes is some basic ingredients and supplies, some of which you probably have already, and you'll have a balanced dinner in no time.

Here are some items you should always have in your Ayurvedic kitchen:

- Legumes (your choice)

- Grains (your choice)

- Organic, local, seasonal vegetables and fruit

- Onions, garlic, ginger

- High-quality sesame and/or coconut oil

- Nuts and seeds according to your Doshic needs

- A rich array of spices and herbs: turmeric, cumin, cinnamon, coriander, asafoetida, cloves, star anise, nutmeg, black pepper, sea salt

- Stevia, monk fruit sweetener, coconut sugar, date sugar, raw honey, or maple syrup (your choice)

And that's it! With these ingredients, you can make any Ayurvedic meal—a healthy grain porridge for breakfast, spiced vegetable curry for lunch, fruit or nuts for a snack, and lentil soup for dinner. You can rotate your ingredients according to the season so you never get bored eating the same thing every day.

> **WISDOM OF THE AGES**
>
> Always have one type of legume and one type of grain on hand. Rotate your vegetables and spices according to the season.

What If You Don't Have the Money?

Cooking Ayurvedically is much more affordable than most other methods of healthy eating. Think about it—what's the most expensive item you end up buying at the grocery store? Usually meat. What's the most affordable? Grains and legumes, especially if you buy them in bulk. The latter are the two main staples of the Ayurvedic diet.

Grains and legumes are packed with protein and healthy carbs, providing all the energy you need. Pair them with vegetables, and you have a complete, balanced meal.

Buying organic can be more expensive than conventional, but you can find local, seasonal vegetables on sale lots of times. Try going to your local farmers' market for great deals.

Meal-planning can save you money, too. Make a schedule of what meals you'll consume every day of the week, and shop accordingly. That way, you only buy what you need. You also can see what's on sale at your local supermarket and plan your meals accordingly. So much food goes to waste today, and you can easily avoid that with some mindful preparation.

Do You Need to Buy Totally Organic?

Ayurveda recommends eating food in their most natural state, but not every food absolutely needs to be organic. If your budget is tight, spend your money on those organic ingredients whose skin you eat. These are the "dirty dozen," the 12 most pesticide-contaminated foods you always should buy organically to avoid the potential toxins in the skin. They are:

- Strawberries
- Spinach
- Nectarines
- Apples
- Peaches
- Pears
- Potatoes
- Cherries
- Grapes
- Celery
- Tomatoes
- Bell Peppers

As a general rule, always buy organic for foods you eat the skin, such as strawberries. Foods that have a skin you remove generally have a lower pesticide load, though not always the case.

The foods with the lowest pesticide content are called the "clean 15." They are:

- Sweet corn
- Avocados
- Pineapples
- Cabbage
- Onions
- Sweet peas (frozen)
- Papayas
- Asparagus

- Mangoes
- Eggplants
- Honeydew melons
- Kiwifruits
- Cantaloupe
- Cauliflower
- Grapefruit

Ideally, choose organic grains and legumes as well because they are often sprayed with pesticides.

Buy as much organic as you can afford, and don't be hard on yourself if you can't purchase all organic items. It's still better to eat nonorganic lentils than junk food.

What If You Don't Have Time to Cook Every Day?

An Ayurvedic diet requires minimal preparation. If you know how to boil water, you know how to make grains and beans. Just soak them beforehand, boil them in water, and enjoy your meal! Later in this chapter, I share some appliances and equipment that can make your cooking time even faster and easier.

Traditional Ayurvedic texts do recommend cooking every day so your food is as fresh as possible, but it is possible to prepare ahead certain things. For example, you can make a large amount of rice or another grain, store it in your refrigerator, and sauté it with various vegetables and oil for dinner. That way, you won't have to make rice from scratch for each meal but still cook the vegetables fresh.

> **WISDOM OF THE AGES**
>
> Ayurveda does not recommend eating leftovers because they are *tamasic* or dull in energy. Freshly cooked food is highest in *prana*, lifeforce.

If you absolutely do not have time, you can prepare a large batch of food and eat the leftovers for the next few days. Just be sure to reheat your meals on the stove, not the microwave, which can damage foods' nutrients.

How Do You Cook for Your Family of Different Doshas?

This is a common question. Not everyone in your family will be the same Dosha, although you may notice some similarities. That doesn't mean you have to make each person his or her own dish. By including the six tastes, each family member can customize his or her own meal to make it fit their unique Doshic needs.

If you have a Vata member of the family, include some warm, cooked root vegetables and grains at every meal. Offer extra ginger and spices they can add to their meals to make them more warming. Keep raw foods separate.

If you have a Pitta family member, keep the chili and other heating spices to the side for the other Doshas to add to their own meals. Avoid using excess garlic in your cooking, and keep nightshade vegetables to the side.

If you have a Kapha member, avoid using too much oil in your cooking. Offer dairy products on the side for other family members to add if they choose. Have extra chili, ginger, and other heating spices on the side for Kaphas.

Many spices and herbs work for all three Doshas, including ginger, turmeric, asafoetida, coriander, and cumin. Spice your food mildly, and offer extra on the side for each person to add more if they choose.

It's also important to include the six tastes (sweet, sour, salty, bitter, pungent, and astringent) at every meal so Doshas can consume the tastes they need more of. The recipes in Chapter 17 work for all three Doshas.

Additionally, Doshas change with the season so you'll have some similarity within your family. In the winters, everyone will need more warming foods, and in the summers, everyone will need more cooling foods. You all live in the same place, so what's seasonal and local is the same for all of you. This removes a lot of the guesswork because your Vikrutis may be more similar than you think.

Keep in mind that Doshic constitutions run in the family. If you are a Vata, you probably have one parent or child who is as well. Your Prakriti, the Doshic constitution you were born with, is based on your DNA, so you'll notice similarities among your family.

Rather than stressing about the things each Dosha is supposed to eat, focus on eliminating the things they're *not* supposed to eat that aren't necessary for any other Dosha. To prepare a tridoshic meal (meaning it works with all three Doshas), avoid raw foods, excess spice, and dairy products, which throw Vata, Pitta, and Kapha off balance, respectively. Roasted vegetables, quinoa, rice, beans, lentils, and other staples can make many appearances on your dinner table. Rotate with the season, include the six tastes, and your job is done!

> ### WISDOM OF THE AGES
>
> Cooking Ayurvedically for different family members is easier than you might think. Prepare a simple vegetable dish of what's available at the farmers' market, and sauté it in digestive-enhancing Ayurvedic spices and herbs. Pair it with some legumes and grains, and you are good to go.

Can You Eat Meat?

Ayurveda does not recommend consuming meat unless necessary to sustain your life. Meat was not recommended for healthy individuals for a number of reasons. Animal proteins are difficult for the body to digest because they contains no enzymes to facilitate with digestion. Subsequently, meat is extremely heavy and often sits in your gastrointestinal tract undigested. This creates toxicity, called ama, which spreads throughout your body, causing a range of imbalances. Meat is extremely acidic, as well, which makes your body more prone to diseases such as cancer. Studies published in the *International Journal of Cancer, Nutrition and Cancer,* and *Cancer* scientific journals have concluded that countries with a higher intake of animal products have higher incidences of breast cancer.

The only times Ayurveda recommends meat consumption is if you suffer from a debilitating disease, such as an autoimmune disorder, extreme fatigue, or an eating disorder, or are a warrior, meaning you exhaust yourself physically. If you are a Vata individual, eating a little bit of animal proteins once a week or month may be enough for your needs. Listen to your body when making the decision.

If you choose to consume meat, be sure it is organic, grass fed, and sustainably sourced. You eat whatever the animal ate, so if it was fed GMO corn and antibiotics, you'll be taking that in as well. That can lead to digestive disorders and other illnesses. According to science news, at least 80 percent of U.S. feedlot cattle are injected with hormones, and an astonishing 80 percent of all antibiotics sold in the United States are used on livestock.

Can You Drink Alcohol?

Ayurveda does not recommend alcohol consumption with the exception of herbalized wine. These wines are called *asavas* and *arishtas* and are medicinal preparations of herbs fermented in jaggary, raw cane sugar, for a specific amount of time. The wine undergoes a fermentation process, making it 5 to 10 percent alcoholic. These preparations are considered medicinal and not for recreational consumption, and the recommended amount is only 4 to 6 teaspoons after meals.

All other types of alcohol are not recommended by Ayurveda and in fact, are called a poison that will bring misery. The Charaka Samhita states, "Those who are unwise and ignorant, who are imbalanced, consider the taking of alcohol to be a creator of happiness; these people lose happiness and purity of mind. The wrong use of alcohol will cause illusion, fear, grief, anger, death and disease. If the memory of our true unbounded nature is impaired, then misery will follow. The wise, acquainted with these adverse effects, avoid alcohol." This basically means imbalanced people who drink alcohol will face negative side effects, and balanced people will know about these side effects and not want to drink alcohol.

Alcohol is dehydrating, full of sugar, acidic, and bad for your digestive system. You can replace it with a stimulating ginger tea to get that same buzz without the negative side effects.

If it's absolutely necessary for you to drink alcohol, the Charaka Samhita states, "If one takes alcohol it must be used in relation to understanding the qualities of the food or drink and the consumer's age, the strength of digestion, current state of health or disease, and season of the year or even time of day." If you do drink, be sure you come to the situation in a good mood, not using alcohol as a means of escape or coping.

Pay attention to your Dosha, and be sure the alcohol will help you remain in balance. Vatas should try a sweet, heating red wine; Pittas should favor a cooling white wine; and Kaphas should have a dry red wine.

> **WISDOM OF THE AGES**
>
> Remember to drink hot water with the wine to prevent dehydration, and make it only a once-in-a-while affair.

How Can You Eat Ayurvedically at a Restaurant?

Although you may face some challenges finding Ayurveda-approved options at restaurants, it is possible. You just have to take some initiative to be sure the restaurant cooks according to your taste (and health).

It helps to hop online and study the restaurant's menu, if it's available. That way, you can see what types of foods are offered, think about how you might make something work for your Dosha, and plan second or third options if your first choice doesn't work out.

At the restaurant, ask for hot water with lemon to aid your digestion. Avoid the ice water restaurants commonly often serve.

WISDOM OF THE AGES

Look to see if the menu has a vegetarian section. If it does, you're in luck. Look for a "Buddha bowl" type dish that contains a variety of the six tastes, such as grains, roasted vegetables, legumes and herbs. If not, look for any vegetable curries or steamed vegetables dishes with grains. Lentil, pumpkin, butternut, black bean or other vegetable and legume soups are also great options, as long as you avoid the heavy cream.

Salads are not recommended in Ayurveda because they are so cooling and difficult to digest. However, they can be consumed in moderation if they have warming ingredients like roasted squash and grains. Pittas can favor more raw foods than the other Doshas.

However, just because something is vegetarian doesn't make it healthy. Many vegetarian dishes contain dairy products, such as cheese-topped salads or buttery vegetables. Be sure to ask what type of oil is used and steer clear from vegetable oils such as canola, corn, soybean, sunflower or safflower oil.

While coconut and olive oil can be extracted by pressing, the vegetable oils mentioned above are unnaturally processed and heated at such high temperatures that they oxidize and become rancid before you even buy them. This oxidization has been linked to cancer, heart disease, endrometrosis, PCOS and other diseases.

Vegetable oils are also processed with a petroleum solvent to extract the oils and treated with chemicals to improve the color and deodorize the harsh smell from the chemical process. Many contain BHA and BHT to keep food from spoiling, which also produce cancerous compounds in the body and have been linked to immune system issues, infertility, behavioral disorders, and liver and kidney damage. They have a very high concentration of Omega 6 to Omega-3 fatty acid ratio, which has also been linked to cancer and other disorders.

WISDOM OF THE AGES

Don't fall for "vegetable oils" as a natural source of fat. Instead, favor coconut, sesame, olive, grapeseed or avocado oil, as well as ghee for non-vegans.

If there's no substantial vegetarian entrée, order two or three sides of cooked vegetables as your entrée. Most restaurants have steamed spinach, brussels sprouts, bok choy, or other vegetable side dishes. Specify that they use one of the approved oils and not too much.

Want something a little more creative? Make a request! Chefs sometimes are delighted to make something off menu if you ask nicely and explain your limitations. Request a dish that's totally plant-based if the chef is amiable. You may be surprised by what he or she comes up with!

> **WISDOM OF THE AGES**
>
> More and more vegetarian and vegan restaurants are opening around the world, making only dishes free of animal products. You can find a list of them at HappyCow (happycow.net). This has saved me on many vacations! Vegan/vegetarian restaurants tend to have more natural, plant-based options with less oil, fried foods, and starches than other restaurants.

What Time Should Your Last Meal of the Day Be?

Ayurveda recommends waiting at least 3 hours, if not longer, after finishing your last meal to sleep. As the sun goes down, so does your digestive fire. You can't break down your food as well at night, which means it sits undigested in your gut, leading to toxicity.

Make lunch your biggest meal of the day, when the sun is high in the sky and your digestive fire is active. That way, you have the rest of the day to burn off the meal. Have a light dinner around 6 P.M. when the sun is setting, and take a gentle walk outside afterward. Then prepare for bed, and head to sleep by 10 P.M.

Questions About Preparing for an Ayurvedic Diet

Now that you know the ins and outs of the an Ayurvedic diet, let's help you prepare. With just a few simple essentials, you'll have all the supplies and ingredients you need to heal your body the Ayurvedic way. You may already have most of them in your kitchen.

Where Should You Start?

Start right where you are! When learning about a new way of eating, it's all too easy to throw yourself right in to it … and then just as quickly fall off the bandwagon, back to where you began.

This is where Ayurveda differs from a diet. A diet is a short-term method of eating for a goal, often weight loss. Ayurveda is a way of life that encompasses eating but includes so much more. Ayurveda merely gives suggestions but does not have strict rules that must be applied. The purpose of Ayurveda is not to lose weight or get fit, although that may happen as a side effect of becoming healthier. It's intention is to help you achieve mind-body balance. Food is a means of getting there because you cannot achieve balance when you aren't physically and mentally sound.

Each week, pick one thing you'd like to integrate into your lifestyle. For example:

> **Week 1:** Eliminate alcohol, tobacco, and coffee from your diet.
>
> **Week 2:** Eat a warming breakfast of cooked grains and spices or stewed apples.

Week 3: Include more of the six tastes in your diet, especially the ones you may be lacking in, such as bitter and astringent.

Week 4: Pack your lunch, and make it the biggest meal of your day. Try another Ayurvedic recipe from my website eatfeelfresh.com.

Week 5: Try following the Doshic daily rhythms, sleeping and rising earlier. Cook another new Ayurvedic recipe.

Week 6: Begin scraping your tongue in the morning, noticing the sticky white ama buildup and signs of what Dosha your tongue is. Make a detoxifying bitter or astringent Ayurvedic recipe.

Week 7: Start a dry brushing and abhyanga self-oil massage practice. Notice how much smoother your body feels and how much calmer your mind is.

Week 8: Try oil pulling for at least 2 minutes. Increase the length you can keep the oil in your mouth over the coming weeks. Use sesame or coconut oil, depending on your Dosha.

Week 9: Give nasal cleaning a shot with a neti pot and nasya nasal cleansing. You'll benefit from a little nose love.

Week 10: By now you should be an Ayurvedic pro. Notice what food grows locally, and get creative in the kitchen. Stock up on more spices, and invite your friends and family over for an Ayurvedic dinner.

In just 10 weeks, you've changed your diet and lifestyle without ever having to throw yourself into a rigid, difficult-to-follow diet.

> **WISDOM OF THE AGES**
>
> Instead of completely abandoning your old diet and devoting yourself to a life of turmeric, go gradually. Make one thing a habit before adding something else. That way, you'll increase your chances of a successful new lifestyle.

Ayurveda is not about extremes. It's about gradual shifts in the right direction. If you can do one positive thing for your mind and body every week, you've had a productive week.

Instead of focusing on how much you can accomplish, focus on how much you can care for yourself. The more you love your mind, body, and spirit, the more you'll be able to achieve in the long run because it will come from a state of balance. You are your greatest project; be sure you give yourself the time and effort you deserve.

What Cooking Equipment Do You Need?

The cooking supplies necessary for an Ayurvedic diet are quite simple. Dehydrators, fancy kitchen tools, expensive blenders, an assortment of chef's knives, and other pricey appliances are not required. You only need the basics: a stove, pots and pans, wooden spoons, a good knife, a cutting board, a soup ladle, and glass containers.

Ayurveda is an ancient system that began before electric refrigerators and ovens even existed. In Ayurvedic times, people would just pick fresh vegetables, herbs, and spices from their farms and cook them in a big pot over a fire. Most of the recipes were designed to be made in a single pot.

Today we have some more advanced tools that can make the process quicker and easier, especially if you're on a tight schedule. Two tools I would recommend are slow cookers, which slowly cook your meals even when you aren't home, and rice cookers, which quickly cook your meal in a fraction of the time.

A slow cooker is extremely useful if you are away from home during the day. Prepare the ingredients in the morning, add them to the slow cooker, set it, and go to work. When you get home, you'll have a freshly cooked meal ready to devour. Many slow cookers have a "warm" mode that keeps the food warm after cooking so it is ready to eat whenever you are. Slow cookers also have the benefit of cooking food at a lower temperature to retain its nutrients. It is actually more similar to the ancient Ayurvedic way of cooking, where food was slowly cooked over the fire for many hours.

Whereas slow cookers are designed to gradually bring your food to the correct temperature, rice cookers cook your food as fast as possible. If you are someone who likes to throw together something off the top of your head based on your current craving, a rice cooker may be a good option for you. Despite the name, rice cookers cook more than just rice. Rice cookers can quickly cook your grains, stews, soups, or even steamed vegetables so they're ready to eat in the shortest amount of time. Rice cookers don't provide the same nutritional benefits and savory flavor as slow cookers, but they work great for a quick meal in fewer than 20 minutes. Some rice cookers also keep the meal warm after heating.

WISDOM OF THE AGES

If you prefer to plan your meal ahead and come home to a freshly cooked meal, get a slow-cooker. If you are a spontaneous chef and want your meal as fast and simple as possible, get a rice or pressure cooker.

I also recommend you have two stainless-steel pots—a larger one for stews, curries, and one-pot dishes, and a smaller one for reheating individual portions. As you cook more, you can purchase other sizes as needed.

Stainless-steel sauté pans are also handy. You can use a large one to sauté a bunch of vegetables at once, a medium one to cook some tofu or brown an onion, and a small one to quickly reheat an individual portion. Many stores sell sets with all three sizes.

You don't need an entire chef's knife set for cooking Ayurvedically, but I do recommend you have two good knives—a 10-inch chef's knife for chopping vegetables and a smaller, 6-inch knife for peeling and cutting little items. These two knives will become your best friends.

No knife is complete without a chopping board. I recommend getting the largest wood chopping board you can fit in your cabinet. That way, you can cut a bunch of vegetables without them falling off your board and making a mess. I prefer wood chopping boards over plastic to prevent bisphenol A (BPA) contamination possible with plastics.

Wooden spoons are another kitchen must-have for stirring stews, tasting stir-fries, and mixing soups. Choose wood over metal because metal can get hot while you cook whereas wood does not.

A metal soup ladle is perfect for doling out freshly made soups. It also makes it easier to scoop out individual portions than trying to tilt the pot and spilling your soup everywhere (not like I'm speaking from experience …).

> **WISDOM OF THE AGES**
>
> A grater is an Ayurvedic kitchen essential because fresh ginger and turmeric are such a large part of the diet. Freshly grating your spices yields much more medicinal benefits and also gives your food an aromatic flavor dried versions simply can't provide. Choose a small, fine grater so you don't get big chunks of ginger in your food (although you might enjoy that!).

Measuring cups and spoons are essential for re-creating recipes and ensuring you have the portions correct. You don't want your curry to be way too spicy because you didn't measure correctly.

A blender or food processor is great if you like making blended soups. In Ayurvedic times, people mashed their soups by hand, so that's always an option if you have the time and really want to go the ancient way. Otherwise, throw your veggies in a blender or food processor and you'll have a bowl of creamy soup in seconds. These days blenders and food processors are relatively inexpensive and will pay for themselves with all the delicious bowls of easy-to-digest roasted vegetable soup they'll help you make.

Last but not least, get some glass containers to store food. Avoid plastic containers because of the risk of BPA contamination, especially because most Ayurvedic food is hot, causing the plastic to leak and release toxins.

Eating Ayurvedically is easy, affordable, healthy, and socially conscious. You don't need a chef's kitchen, tons of equipment, or all the time in the world to follow a more Ayurvedic diet. All you really need is the basics, both in terms of supplies and ingredients, to give your body the gift of balance.

The Least You Need to Know

- To stock your Ayurvedic kitchen, all you really need is some legumes, grains, vegetables, oils, and spices.
- To cook for family members of different Doshas, make a basic meal of cooked seasonal vegetables in various preparations, from soups to stews to curries. Avoid raw foods, spices, and dairy to avoid unbalancing Vatas, Pittas, and Kaphas, respectively.
- When dining out, look to the vegetarian options, soups without cream, and vegetable side dishes. Ask for less oil in your meal when ordering, and seek out vegan and vegetarian restaurants wherever you go for healthier options.
- Some basic kitchen equipment will prepare you for cooking Ayurvedically: pots, pans, wooden spoons, knives, cutting board, and glass containers. A slow cooker or rice cooker can make preparation quicker and easier, too.

The Spiritual Side of Ayurveda

What brings many people to Ayurveda are the physical benefits; what makes them stay are the spiritual benefits. In Part 5, we look at the three cosmic forces, universal qualities, and the energies we are all made of. You may be familiar with your physical body (I hope you are!), but in this part, I show you that you actually have four more. Curious yet? I also discuss chakras, koshas, and everything in between, bringing you back into your true state: bliss.

CHAPTER 19

Cosmic Forces and Universal Qualities

You're well versed on the three Doshas—Vata, Pitta, and Kapha. You know the five elements they're comprised of, the foods they're related to, and how they affect your seven bodily tissues. Now I'm going to show you *why* you need to seek balance in the first place. The purpose of balance is to tap into your inner bliss.

What makes Ayurveda so unique is that it is a spiritual science. It connects the seen and the unseen, the physical and the metaphysical. In this chapter, we move into the subtler side of Ayurveda and the effects of your diet and lifestyle on your spirit. We explore the three cosmic forces of Ayurveda—ojas, tejas, and prana, which are subtle forces of Kapha, Pitta, and Vata. I also discuss the three universal qualities that can be used to describe all things—*sattva* (light), *rajas* (movement), and *tamas* (darkness).

In This Chapter

- The three cosmic forces of Ayurveda
- Ways to regain luster, passion, and flow in your life
- The three universal qualities in everything and everyone
- The spiritual side effects of onions and garlic

The Three Cosmic Forces

Just like there are three Doshas—Vata, Pitta, and Kapha—there are three cosmic forces—*ojas, tejas,* and *prana,* which are the subtler forms of each Dosha. By "subtler form," I mean how it affects you on a more spiritual level.

Ojas is connected to the Kapha Dosha, tejas is connected to the Pitta Dosha, and Prana is connected to the Vata Dosha. Ojas is expressed as vitality, endurance, fertility, and patience, all qualities of Kapha. Tejas is expressed as courage, intellect, drive, and radiance, all qualities of Pitta. Prana is expressed as creativity, lightness, enthusiasm, and intuition, all qualities of Vata. You have (and need) all three vital essences within you.

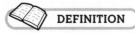 **DEFINITION**

Ojas is the subtle essence related to health and well-being. It makes you peaceful and patient. **Tejas** is the essence related to radiance and glow. It makes you intelligent and courageous. **Prana** is the essence related to vital life force and breath. It makes you flexible and creative. You require all three vital essences to be balanced.

Let's explore each cosmic force, study the signs of their balance and imbalance, and learn what to do if yours is depleted.

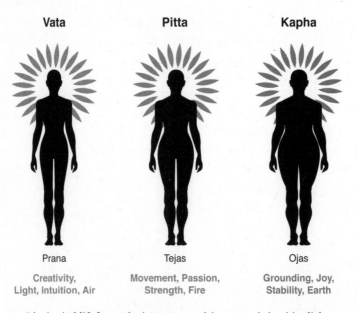

Vata	Pitta	Kapha
Prana	Tejas	Ojas
Creativity, Light, Intuition, Air	Movement, Passion, Strength, Fire	Grounding, Joy, Stability, Earth

Ojas is vital life force; tejas is courageous drive; prana is intuitive light.

Ojas: The Luster of Life

Have you ever seen a person who just radiated with life? They seemed to glow from within, shining out like golden light. That's ojas.

Ojas is the subtle essence related to health, vitality, immunity, and well-being. It results from proper digestion and forms your bodily tissues, organs, skin, and cells. That's why digestion is so important in Ayurveda. The better your digestion, the more ojas you have.

Healthy Ojas

Signs of healthy ojas include glowing skin, peaceful energy, high stress tolerance, and strong immune system.

Ojas is stored in the heart, and people high in ojas are heart-centered people who can easily connect with themselves and others around them. They are giving, charitable, and patient. People are naturally drawn to those with healthy ojas because just being in their presence feels warming and delightful. I like to compare ojas to the sun—radiant, vibrant, and always shining no matter the weather. People high in ojas are stable and centered, able to easily deal with stress and disturbances.

> **WISDOM OF THE AGES**
>
> Ojas gives you a radiant glow that naturally attracts people to your peaceful energy.

Low Ojas

How does ojas get weak? There are a number of ways, and they all relate to digestion, both of food and emotions:

- Over-, under-, binge, or emotional eating
- Consuming processed foods, meat, sugar, and cheese
- Eating stale, canned, or frozen meals
- Physical trauma
- Chronic illness or pain
- Excess travel
- Lack of sleep
- Aging
- Alcohol, smoking, drugs
- Jealousy, anger, hatred, fear
- Stress/overwork
- Emotional trauma

As you can see, it's just as important for your thoughts to be as healthy as your diet because they both can deplete ojas. If you eat too much, too little, the wrong foods, or toxins, your body suffers. If you compare yourself to others, hold grudges, or live in a constant state of worry, your mind suffers. Eventually, an imbalance in one affects the other.

Signs of weak ojas include dull skin, lethargy, depression, anxiety, constant illness, eating disorders, and emaciation. If this sounds like you, it's very important that you regain ojas to feel alive again.

How to Regain Ojas

To return your ojas to balance, the number-one thing you have to do is heal your digestion. Avoid processed, frozen, and canned foods; refined sugar and carbs; meat; and other ingredients that will throw off your balance. Instead, consume more *sattvic* foods, which are simple, plant-based ingredients like grains, cooked vegetables, fresh fruit, nuts, and seeds. Include the six tastes in your diet as well, and eat mindfully. Take care of your body, and practice meditation.

The following foods help increase your ojas:

- Avocados
- Coconut products
- Dates
- Fresh fruit
- Ghee and raw milk

- Grains
- Healthy oils
- Nuts and seeds
- Sweet potatoes
- Turmeric

Much of ojas is emotional. To bring back your life force, do more of the things you love, such as:

- Take a walk in nature.
- Attend a dance class.
- Spend time with animals and children.
- Practice yoga, pranayama, or tai chi.
- Create art.
- Write in a journal.

- Cook a delicious meal.
- Meditate.
- Oil your body.
- Take a warm bath.
- Read a book.
- Redecorate your house.
- Make a vision board.

Release thoughts that are no longer serving you. Let go of any anger or attachment you have to the past. Allow yourself to surrender to the present moment. Make your home your sanctuary so you truly love where you live. All these little things help you rebuild your ojas.

Ojas-Enhancing Tonic

Creamy almonds pair with sweet cardamom, cinnamon, rose and saffron in this warming recipe that rejuvenates your ojas, replenishing your vital life force. This recipe is similar to a make your own almond milk except you don't need a nut milk bag.

10 almonds	$1/2$ tsp. ground cinnamon
2 cups water	1 TB. rose petals
$1/2$ tsp. cardamom	1 pinch saffron

1. Soak almonds in water overnight.

2. Drain almonds and peel off skin. They'll come right off once soaked.

3. Add almonds to a blender with two cups water and blend until smooth. Add cardamom, cinnamon, rose petals and saffron and blend again.

4. Pour beverage into a small saucepan over medium high heat and cover until starting to bubble but not boiling. Enjoy as a nightly tonic.

This recipe will give you a healthy glow, improve your immune system, and prevent aging and disease by replenishing your ojas. You'll also feel a sense of calmness by having this drink. It's best for Vatas and Pittas, as it increases Kapha.

Tejas: The Spark of Radiance

Whereas ojas promotes a peaceful energy, tejas ignites the fire underneath it all. You've probably met a person who's just on fire—they're confident, powerful, and radiant from within. There is a certain twinkle in their eyes that shows their inner light. They seem to glow, and people naturally tend to follow them. That's tejas.

Tejas is the subtle essence related to strength, longevity, intelligence, luster, and color. It gives you bright and shiny eyes, luminous skin, and a brilliant mind. It's the potential energy of fire and light.

Healthy Tejas

Signs of healthy tejas include a radiant personality, bright eyes, sharp mind, decisiveness, strong leadership abilities, and bravery.

Tejas is related to your digestive fire and metabolism. Those with too much tejas may have Pitta imbalance symptoms such as hyperacidity and heartburn. Those with too little may have weak digestion and sluggish metabolism.

> **WISDOM OF THE AGES**
>
> Tejas gives you a passionate zest that allows you to think and lead with precision and strength.

Low Tejas

How does tejas weaken? Anything that causes burnout weakens your tejas:

- Overexertion
- Overheating
- Overexercise
- Physical and emotional trauma
- Stress
- Anger
- Alcohol, smoking, drugs

Anything that imbalances Pitta also imbalances tejas because they are both related to the fire element. It's important to kindle your flame without exhausting it to keep your tejas balanced.

Signs of weak tejas include a lackluster mind; indecisiveness; fear; dull eyes and skin; lack of passion, purpose, or creativity; trouble learning new things; poor leadership skills; inability to concentrate; and stubbornness. If this sounds like you, you must regain your tejas to reclaim your radiance.

How to Regain Tejas

To bring your tejas back into balance, you'll have to stimulate your internal fire to bring heat to your subtle body:

- Practice breath of fire: short, quick, and firm inhales and exhales through your nose.
- Solar pranayama: slowly breathe in through your right nostril and out through your left nostril for 5 minutes.
- Increase spices in your diet, especially ginger, cumin, and chile peppers.
- Exercise more rigorously to get your body moving and your blood flow going.
- Set goals for yourself such as finishing a book or completing a project.
- Gaze into a candle flame to increase your fire energy.

Tejas-Boosting Tonic

Need a kick to power through your day? This tejas-boosting tonic is packed with pungent ginger and cayenne, balanced with sour lemon and sweet honey, bringing your passionate and purpose-driven Pitta energy up.

2 cups water	$^1/_2$ tsp. cayenne
1 (1-in.) piece ginger, peeled and grated (1 TB.)	Juice of $^1/_2$ lemon
	1 tsp. raw honey or maple syrup

1. In a small pan over medium high heat, bring water to a boil.

2. Add ginger and cayenne, and steep for at least 10 minutes.

3. Add lemon juice and raw honey or maple syrup, and enjoy as a stimulating beverage to stoke your internal tejas flame.

This tonic is useful for days when you feel like you need an extra energy boost to get you through the day or your digestion feels weak and slow. It also stimulates the metabolism and is most recommended for Kapha types, though Vatas can also benefit as long as it's not too spicy.

Prana: The Vital Life Force

If you've ever practiced yoga, you may have heard the term *prana*. Prana is the breath of life, comprised of the air element. It is responsible for movement, respiration, circulation, and oxygenation and governs all things related to your mind, thoughts, and emotions. Although you cannot see it, you always feel it. If you've ever felt a sense of stillness while chanting "Om" or had a sudden rush of butterflies when life just seemed to be falling into place, that's prana moving through you.

Prana is felt most in your breath. When you still your mind, you can tune in to the more subtle layers of your body, tapping into the endless source of inspiration that exists within you.

Healthy Prana

Signs of healthy prana include enthusiasm, life force, creativity, adaptability, energy, and motivation.

Prana is located in your brain's hypothalamus. It sends out signals to your sympathetic and parasympathetic nervous system as well as your intercostal muscles and diaphragm. This is why your breath is so connected to your emotions.

When you take in a breath, your intercostal muscles contract and your diaphragm moves downward. This increases space in your chest cavity, causing your lungs to expand. When you breathe out, your diaphragm relaxes and moves upward, causing your intercostal muscles to relax, making the space in your chest cavity smaller. You aren't consciously thinking about this movement, but your brain is constantly signaling your lungs to inhale and exhale, keeping you alive. This is all thanks to prana.

> **WISDOM OF THE AGES**
>
> According to Ayurveda, your soul, or *atman,* is reflected in your breath. The deeper your breathing, the more you can connect to your true nature. The space of absolute stillness between your inhales and exhales is meditation. (More on breathing during meditation later in this chapter.)

Prana governs your emotions, which are also held in your lungs. Notice how your breath changes when you're angry and stressed versus when you're calm and peaceful. When you are in a state of distress, you take short, shallow breaths. This triggers your parasympathetic nervous system's fight-or-flight response, and your brain immediately gets the signal that there's a threat and releases cortisol, the stress hormone. This is prana at work. Your breath indicates to your nervous system, which indicates to your brain that things are not safe. Your entire being feels restless.

When you are peaceful, your breathing slows down. You take deeper and slower breaths, pausing between each inhale and exhale. Your parasympathetic nervous system decides there's no need to worry and goes into a state of rest. As a result, your mind releases serotonin, the happiness hormone.

Many studies, such as one published in the *Archives of General Psychiatry,* confirm that mindfulness-based cognitive therapy (MBCT) "offers protection against relapse/recurrence on a par with that of maintenance antidepressant pharmacotherapy." Simply the effect of becoming more mindful of your breath in any situation shifts your attention away from the stressful situation, reducing your risk of depression.

> **WISDOM OF THE AGES**
>
> Prana allows circulation of energy by utilizing the subtle power of your own breath.

Low Prana

How does prana become weak? When your emotions are negative:

- Stressful situations
- Emotional or physical trauma
- Longing for the past
- Jealous, anger, comparison

- Hatred, fear, anxiety
- Chronic illness
- Excess caffeine
- Poor breathing

Notice that everything comes back to your breath. Any situation that causes you to take short, shallow breaths depletes your prana.

Signs of low prana include shortness of breath, low energy, constriction in the body, coldness or numbness in the extremities, excess worrying or anxiety, and energy depletion. If this sounds like you, it's very important to recover your prana to find happiness again.

How to Regain Prana

If you can breathe, you can enhance your prana. All it takes is reclaiming your breath, which is the key to life. Meditation is one of the best ways to get back in touch with your breathing. Meditation is an approach to training your mind to be still. Just like you have to exercise your muscles to become fit, you must practice meditation to increase your awareness.

Meditation does not mean you have to sit quietly and think of nothing. In fact, the more you tell yourself not to think about anything, the more your mind will race. The easiest way to meditate is just to focus on your breath. That way, you have something to concentrate on to prevent your mind from wandering.

Here's one of my favorite meditation practices. You can use it to increase your pranic life force:

1. Sit comfortably in a chair or cross-legged on the floor, however you're comfortable. (I don't recommend lying down because you could fall asleep.)

2. Close your eyes and take a deep inhale in and then an audible exhale out. Repeat, letting all the stagnant air exit your lungs.

3. When you feel like you've released tension, bring your attention to your breath. Notice how you breathe naturally. Don't try to change your breath. Simply observe it.

4. Notice the movement of your body as you breathe in. Feel how your rib cage expands as your lungs fill with air and how your chest and shoulders collapse as you breathe out.

5. Continue paying attention to your breath. You may notice that your breathing has slowed down. Continue breathing, totally breathing out all the air in your lungs before taking a new breath in.

6. As you continue breathing, gradually try to increase the space of stillness between your inhales and your exhales.

Congratulations! You just meditated.

As you can see, meditation doesn't have to be an elaborate practice. You don't need to be a meditation master to benefit from simple breathing practices. All it takes is a few minutes of connecting with your breath every day to reap the immense benefits of meditation.

> **WISDOM OF THE AGES**
>
> For 5 minutes every morning and 5 minutes every night, practice meditation to transition between a sleeping and waking state. You'll notice immediately how much more clear your mind is for the rest of the day when you wake up and meditate instead of checking your email. You'll also sleep much better when you've taken a few moments to silence your mind instead of staring into the blue light of your cellphone screen. See if you can add an extra minute to your meditation practice every week.

The Three Universal Qualities

Mother Nature is a magnificent, multifaceted, and moody mama. Sometimes she amazes us with her tranquility and stillness, more beautiful than the most talented artist's creation. At other times, she is rough and wild, stirring up hurricanes and earthquakes. Then there are times when she is dense and heavy, such as on rainy days or during snow storms.

Ayurveda classifies the three qualities of nature as *sattva, rajas,* and *tamas.* Sattva is pure, like a picture-perfect sunny day. Rajas is intense, like an approaching tornado. Tamas is dark, like a never-ending storm. These three qualities exist not only in nature, but in all things and people as well. These qualities are called the *gunas* and are based on the circle of life. All things are born, live, and die. Sattva represents creation, rajas represents maintenance and motion, and tamas represents death and destruction.

In modern Ayurveda, the gunas are used to describe the nature of foods, medicines, and behaviors. They help us understand how a certain ingredient or experience will make us feel. Let's delve deeper into the three gunas and what each represents.

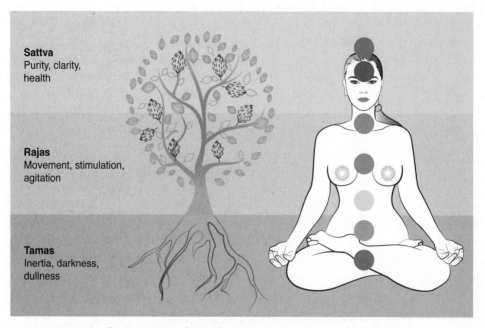

Sattva is related to purity; rajas is related to movement and tamas is related to inertia.

Sattva: The Light of Consciousness

Sattva represents all things good and pure in the world. It evokes qualities of clarity, love, compassion, alertness, and cooperativeness. Sattva is the feeling of waking up in the morning with the energy to take on the day. We all have sattva inside of us and should actively try to seek more. Sattva evokes intelligence, good health, focus, creativity, and lightness in the mind and body. It's similar to the Vata Dosha, but actually all Doshas in balance are sattvic—complete and whole.

Sattvic people are loving, compassionate, honest, energized, generous, spiritually connected, and humble. They are naturally peaceful, creative, and in touch with themselves. They are respectful to others, animals, and nature.

Sattvic foods give your body energy without taxing it. Think of the feeling you have after a good, healthy meal—grounded, energized, and satisfied. That's sattva in action. Mindful eating is considered sattvic.

Examples of sattvic foods include fresh vegetables, juicy fruits, mung beans, certain grains, raw nuts, fresh and raw dairy products, turmeric, ginger, cinnamon, fennel, and cardamom. The sattvic tastes are fresh, light, nourishing, sweet, and juicy. An example of a Sattvic meal is brown rice with steamed seasonal vegetables. You should aim to make most of your meals sattvic because these foods are the foundation to higher states of consciousness.

> **DEFINITION**
>
> **Sattva** represents purity, clarity, and potential energy. It illuminates you with knowledge, wisdom, compassion, and enlightenment. Fresh vegetables, fruit, certain grains, and easily digestible meals are considered sattvic.

Rajas: Kinetic Energy

Rajas represents movement, power, action, pleasure, and pain. It is restless, dominating, and aggressive in energy. You can compare rajas to the Pitta Dosha because it creates transformation, but any Dosha can become rajasic when pushed to the extreme.

Rajasic people are charismatic and skillful speakers and entrepreneurs. However, when they're out of balance, they can be impatient, self-centered, egotistic, and controlling. They are passionate and hard-working but can be jealous and competitive, too. Rajasic people deeply fear failure.

Rajasic foods have a stimulating effect on your mind and body. They include all Pitta-related foods: coffee, caffeinated tea, fermented foods, certain grains and legumes, garlic, onions, nightshades, sour fruit, spicy or salty foods, meat, and eggs. The rajasic tastes are hot, bitter, sour, dry, or salty. Eating in a rush is considered rajasic as well.

Certain rajasic foods can be valuable to the Vata and Kapha Dosha, who may benefit from extra movement and fire in their body. However, Pitta types should avoid rajasic ingredients because they can throw them off balance.

> **DEFINITION**
>
> **Rajas** is invigorating and stimulating, representing movement, passion, and energy. It fills you with power, but excess can lead to aggression. Stimulants, nonvegetarian foods, and pungent tastes are considered rajasic.

Tamas: Inertia

Tamas represents darkness and inactivity. If sattva is sunrise and rajas is the daytime, tamas is the night. In a balanced amount, tamas brings rest and rejuvenation, but in excess, it can make you lazy, tired, and lack self-control.

Everyone has tamas built into their DNA. It provides support and density in the way that Kapha is the building Dosha. If you were always moving and creating, you would not be balanced. However, you have to be sure you are not dominated by tamasic energy or you'll become fatigued, self-indulgent, possessive, and depressed.

Tamasic foods have a sedative effect on the mind and body. Natural foods considered tamasic are onions, garlic, and mushrooms because they're so grounding. Tamasic foods numb pain and were recommended in times of war and distress. They make us more Kapha and grounded, particularly recommended for airy Vata types.

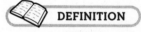

WISDOM OF THE AGES

Onions and garlic are both tamasic and rajasic in energy because they are both stimulating as well as deadening. Garlic is a natural aphrodisiac and is recommended for those with a loss of sex drive, particularly Vatas. Ayurveda recommends moderate amounts of onions and garlic for the Vata Dosha who can benefit from the invigorating and grounding qualities. Kaphas can have small amounts, and Pittas should avoid them. Garlic and onions increase immunity, boost white blood cell count, are antibacterial, and cleanse yeast from the system. However, they also are overly stimulating and can cause agitation, aggression, and dullness for those with excess heat or earth.

Unhealthy tamasic foods include processed foods, frozen or microwaved meals, meat, alcohol, refined sugar, blue cheese, fertilized eggs, tobacco, breads, and pastries. These foods make you feel heavy after consumption and should be totally avoided. Overeating and consuming leftover food is considered tamasic as well.

DEFINITION

Tamas is dark, slow, and dull and evokes qualities of inertia, inactivity, and lethargy. Tamasic foods include processed and frozen meals, refined sugar and carbs, meat, alcohol, onions, and garlic.

Sattva, rajas, and tamas all relate to one another. On one side of the spectrum is sattva, which is pure light, and on the other side is tamas, which is darkness. Rajas moves the forces in either way, depending on what you consume the most of.

Sattva is like the bright idea. However, without rajas, the idea won't come to life, and without rest, you won't be able to recover. Sometimes you have go inward to replenish and become whole again.

The Least You Need to Know

- Three subtle forces are related to the Doshas: ojas, tejas, and prana.
- Ojas is related to Kapha and gives you glowing skin, patience, stability, and immunity.
- Tejas is related to Pitta and provides you with radiant personality, shiny eyes, and a sharp mind.
- Prana is related to Vata and causes creativity, movement, and enthusiasm.
- Three universal qualities relate to all people, places, and things: sattva, rajas, and tamas.
- Sattva evokes purity and health; rajas creates movement and is stimulating; and tamas causes inertia and dullness.

CHAPTER 20

The Koshas:
Your Five Layered Bodies

How many bodies do you have? You'd probably answer just one, the one you can see and feel. According to Ayurveda, however, you actually have five bodies that extend far beyond your physical. These bodies, or layers, are all connected to your deeper soul.

The reason you must work so hard to balance your mind and body is so you can tap into your soul self. Your soul knows exactly what you should be doing and what your purpose here on Earth is. Your soul operates from a place of love, joy, and union. Your soul is your highest self.

In this chapter, you start to understand more about your deeper, soul level so you can tune in and listen to your inner voice of wisdom. I teach you about the deeper layers of your body you never knew about before, and by the end of the chapter, you'll see how interconnected your spiritual, intellectual, energetic, and physical selves truly are.

In This Chapter

- Getting to know your soul self
- Your five bodies—and only one you've seen in the mirror
- The differences among your body, breath, mind, and intuition
- Why underneath it all, we are pure bliss

People Are Human Radios

People are energetic beings. Although they live in human bodies, they have many layers of vibrating energy surrounding them, sending and receiving signals. In a way, people are human radios, constantly picking up on these subtle vibrations. This is why certain people, places, and things give you good or bad vibes.

Even if you don't see these layers, they still exist. Think about it: do you see the sounds coming out of a radio? No, but you still pick up on them. Energy works the same way; it's felt but not seen.

Not only do you give off vibrations, but you are constantly receiving them as well. Your intuition works through these senses, and the more tuned-in you are to the subtle vibrations, the more aligned with your true self you become.

The Five Bodies

Ayurveda categorizes this energetic field into five sheaths, called the *koshas*.

I understand how this might sound a little far-fetched, and you might be thinking *How can I have five bodies when I've only seen one?* You've actually been in contact with your other bodies, almost every day. And by just thinking about this question now, you are in contact with several of them.

Have you ever sensed that you were getting sick right before you did? Your body felt fine, but something within you said "Take extra care of yourself because you may become ill." That was one of the outer layers of your body communicating with one of the inner layers. Your energy detected illness and signaled your mind before it manifested in your body. These were your koshas at work, constantly communicating with one another.

The five koshas are unseen sheaths surrounding your body that sense energy: *annamaya* (sheath of food/physical body), *pranamaya* (sheath of energy/energetic body), *manomaya* (sheath of mind/mental body), *vijnanamaya* (sheath of wisdom/intuitive body), and *anandamaya* (sheath of bliss/blissful body).

> **DEFINITION**
>
> Your **koshas** are five layers surrounding your physical body that comprise your whole being. They are your physical body, energetic body, mental body, intuitive body, and blissful body.

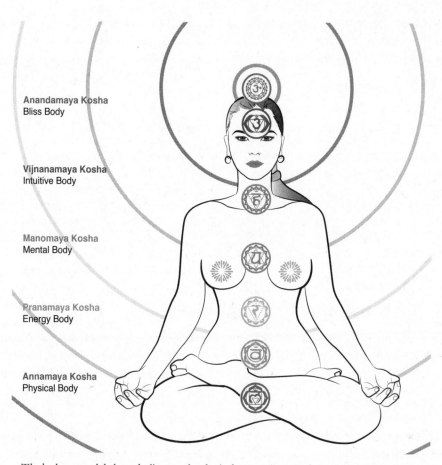

Anandamaya Kosha
Bliss Body

Vijnanamaya Kosha
Intuitive Body

Manomaya Kosha
Mental Body

Pranamaya Kosha
Energy Body

Annamaya Kosha
Physical Body

The koshas, or subtle layer bodies, are the physical, energetic, mental, intuitive and bliss bodies.

Annamaya Kosha (Physical Body)

The *annamaya kosha* is the body you are most familiar with, the one you see in the mirror every day. This is your only tangible body, comprised of skin, bones, muscle, tissues, organs, blood, and water. The term *annamaya* literally means "comprised of food" because remember, you are made up of what you eat.

Your physical body is your most basic form but still of upmost importance. It's the body in which you experience all the others and truly the foundation of your spiritual practice. If you are not physically healthy, you cannot access your more subtle layers. This is why Ayurveda recommends eating healthfully, drinking teas, practicing yoga, sleeping soundly, and spending time outside, among its countless other suggestions. Your first priority is taking care of the temple you reside in so you can experience the bliss of life.

When you are connected to your annamaya kosha, you feel comfortable in your physical body. You exercise, take care of yourself, feel sexually balanced, and have confidence in your body.

When you are disconnected from your annamaya kosha, you disassociate from your physical body. This can cause binge eating, addiction, drinking, drug use, eating disorders, laziness, and self-harm.

Here are some ideas for connecting with your annamaya kosha:

- Eat mindfully, and tune in to your body's needs.

- Practice yoga and meditation.

- Perform abhyanga self-oil massage.

- Move your body in a way that feels good—dance, sports, or other forms of physical activity.

Pranamaya Kosha (Energy Body)

With some people, you just can tell what their energy is like. What you're observing is their *pranamaya kosha*. Your pranic body is your energy and the next thing you notice about another person after their physical body. It's the first sheath surrounding your physical body, about 2½ inches away from you skin. Your pranamaya kosha is also referred to as an "aura" or "etheric" body.

This layer is made up of your pranic life force. Your pranamaya kosha gives off the vibration of how you are breathing. When you are tense and stressed, your breaths are fast and shallow. When you are relaxed and peaceful, your breaths are slow and deep. Just that difference in breath gives off a totally different frequency.

 WISDOM OF THE AGES

> Your Dosha says a lot about how you breathe. Vatas typically breathe quick, shallow, and cool breaths. Pittas breathe hot, shallow, and fiery breaths because of their heat energy. Kaphas breathe slow, deep, and cool breaths.

When your pranamaya kosha is balanced, you are connected to your breath. You have a calming energy and don't easily become frustrated. You can pick up on the vibration of others and are aware of their energies.

When your pranamaya kosha is imbalanced, you are out of touch with your breaths. You may have fast and shallow or hot and heavy inhales and exhalations. You are out of touch with your energy and cannot pick up on others'.

Here's how to connect with your pranamaya kosha:

- Notice your breath. Try to take deeper, slower breaths from your belly.

- Practice pranayama, or controlled breathing.

- Become aware of the subtle energies of everyone and everything around you, from people to trees.

Manomaya Kosha (Mental Body)

"My name is Sahara Rose, and I am an Ayurvedic practitioner and author of *Idiot's Guides: Ayurveda*." That's not me talking—that's my *manomaya kosha*.

Your manomaya kosha is your mental self. This layer contains everything you know, including your sense of self, or ego. Your manomaya kosha is constructed of the things you were taught, the beliefs you hold, and your perception of the world. My body is not Sahara; it's just a body. My energy is not Sahara; it's a vibration. Only in my mind have I decided I am Sahara. It is my mentally constructed sense of self.

Similarly, you are not your body or your mind. You are your soul.

Your soul is different from your personality, which is a construct of your mind. Your personality is the part of yourself that encounters other people in day-to-day life. It's the "Hi, I'm _____, and I like to _____." It carries emotions, attachments, and judgments and learns about the world through comparison and experience.

Your soul, however, is unchanging and ever-knowing. It doesn't go through phases or have mood swings. It's who you truly are on a deeper, core level. It's who you always were and always will be. It was you as a child and will be you the day you die and even beyond that. It is infinite.

Your soul holds the gifts you were put on Earth to do. It contains infinite inspiration, energy, and downloads from the universe. If you've ever had a moment of absolute wisdom, that was your soul speaking.

> **WISDOM OF THE AGES**
>
> Your soul is who you are underneath your personality—the true you that has existed since your childhood and maybe even in past lives before that. By knowing your soul, you will discover your true purpose.

That's not to say your mind is useless. Your mental body is important because it contains knowledge and identity. I wouldn't have been able to write this book if it wasn't for my manomaya kosha. However, many of us become too stuck in our mental selves. We lose association with our physical, energetic, and spiritual bodies and only see ourselves as our egos. This can either make us self-obsessed or anxious because we are living in the mind, not the soul.

Your manomaya kosha contains your accumulated mental patterns. These are the ways you go about leading your life based on your upbringing and experience. We all carry our own stories, which are frameworks through which we see the world. For example, someone who grew up in poverty may have a "there isn't enough" outlook. This causes them to adapt a scarcity mind-set to everything in life, which may cause them to become short sighted and greedy, or even leading them to steal.

Another person may have always sought the approval of their parents and look at life with an "I need the approval of others in order to be happy" philosophy. They may go through life trying to please others before themselves, leading them to make unfulfilling life choices. These mental patterns are called *samskaras*. Your samskaras can hold you back from your true potential. They cause you to see the world from a state of illusion rather than reality. Instead of seeing the opportunities in life, you might focus on the lack of them. Rather than choosing your own path, you might follow the steps of others.

> **WISDOM OF THE AGES**
>
> No one is free of samskaras. Everyone sees the world from their own unique perspective based on their upbringing, cultural conditioning, and years of experiences. However, to drop your stories, you first must become aware of them. Notice the repeated patterns in your life. These contain cues of your own samskaras.

You must become aware of your perceptions in order to become free of them. Letting go of your stories creates a space in your mind for new creative thoughts and infinite possibilities.

When your manomaya kosha is balanced, you feel connected to your mind and sense of self. You are confident, inquisitive, intelligent, and aware. You do not play the role of the victim but instead take ownership of your actions.

When your manomaya kosha is out of balance, you become egotistical and self-obsessed or unconfident and unsure. Your sense of self is either too strong, and you put yourself before others, or too faint, causing weakness and insecurity.

Here are some suggestions for connecting with your manomaya kosha:

- Activate your mind. Write, read, practice puzzles, or do math problems.

- Practice saying "I am" in the mirror.

- Be confident in who you are. Express your divine colors.

- Create art, writing, music, or other forms of your own unique expression.

Vijnanamaya Kosha (Intuitive Body)

After you've removed any blocks in your three lower koshas—your physical, energetic, and mental bodies—you can tap into your higher self.

Have you ever had a deep, wise voice from within you give you perfect advice with absolute clarity … and then moments later wonder where the heck that voice came from? That was your intuition.

The fourth sheath, *vijnanamaya kosha,* is the source of such moments of wisdom. It guides you on your higher path and speaks to you in subtle whispers. If you've ever felt a pull toward a certain direction and that ended up changing your life forever, your vijnanamaya kosha is the one to thank.

The more connected you are with your intuition, the more you receive "downloads" from the universe containing great insight. These downloads are essentially messages of divine wisdom and realization from your higher self. They give you an idea of what you are supposed to be doing and make you more aware of your true nature.

WISDOM OF THE AGES

The universe is constantly communicating with you. The more you can pick up on its subtle energies, the more in line you become with your true nature. By healing your body, enhancing your prana, and releasing your samskaras, you can more finely tune in to this intuitive layer.

In this kosha, you become aware of *buddhi,* the discriminative intellect and knowledge of the ego. You are aware that you aren't your physical body, your thoughts, or even your personality. You are able to recognize your emotions without being attached to them.

Morality lies in this kosha. You realize you have the free will to make decisions in your life. It's up to you to choose what's right. *Yamas* and *niyamas* are ethical rules that tell you to not steal, lie, harm, or overindulge, and these arise from your wisdom body. Most people on a spiritual path are deeply aware of this kosha.

Here are a few ways to connect with your vijnanamaya kosha:

- Realize you are not your ego but the soul beneath it.

- Connect to your higher self for guidance.

- Clear your mind so you can receive downloads from the universe.

- Follow your intuition.

Anandamaya Kosha (Bliss Body)

When you have expanded beyond the koshas, you achieve self-realization. In your truest form, you are a blissful being. Bliss is not a fleeting emotion but rather an absolute experience. You don't witness the bliss but rather become the bliss. How can this be?

Notice the difference between dancing a dance and becoming one with the dance. When you are the dancer, you are merely performing the steps. Your ego is still in place, aware of how you appear, and your mind is still involved, coordinating your moves. When you become one with the dance, there is no more you anymore. You have become one with the rhythm. When the dance and the dancer become one, that is pure bliss.

> **WISDOM OF THE AGES**
>
> Bliss occurs when you are free of your worries, stresses, anxieties, aches, pains, and even your own ego self. It's when there stops being a "you" and you become one with the experience. The singer becomes the song. The artist becomes the painting. The musician becomes the melody. The yogi becomes the asana. The meditator becomes the moment in time. This is true bliss.

Everyone has felt glimpses of this blissfulness before, but true enlightenment is to extend its visitation and bring it forth in your everyday life. How can you feel bliss on a daily basis, leading your ordinary life? Through mind, body, and spirit alignment. Ayurveda, yoga, and meditations are just tools to help you achieve this balance. When you heal your body, slow down your breathing, become aware of your surroundings, let go of your stories, and listen to your intuition, you achieve self-realization.

Here are some pointers on connecting with your anandamaya kosha:

- Participate in an ecstatic dance, a free-flowing silent dance party.

- Practice yoga.

- Try a guided meditation or visualization.

- Play a musical instrument or sing a song.

- Get lost in nature.

Beyond the Koshas People Are One

In their truest beings, people are all the same. There is no separation between you or me or anyone else. People are all just different branches of the same tree, connected to the same trunk, fed the same water, and nourished by the same soil. Rather than comparing one leaf as more green and another as more red, you must realize everyone arises from the same source. The differences between people are merely illusions, preventing them from realizing that they are all one.

According to Ayurveda, every action has an energetic reaction. When you eat a balanced diet, you feel mentally balanced. When you begin your days in meditation, you have more meditative days. When you treat your body with love, more love will show up in all aspects of your life. These little things you do, like soak your beans and dry brush your body, aren't just so you win the Ayurvedic lottery. It's so your body and mind are no longer obstacles preventing you from accessing your deeper soul self.

In your core being, you are pure bliss. Bliss is not momentary. It isn't being drunk from wine or indulging in a chocolate cake. Those are just moments of satisfaction, only temporary illusions. True bliss is everlasting and results when your body, mind, and spirit are connected.

The whole purpose of seeking health is so you can tap into this higher, awakened side of yourself. This internal consciousness operates from a place of joy, truth, awareness, and love. It is the wisdom that guides you through life's questions and turbulences.

Everything in Ayurveda is a tool to help you get to this very state of pure bliss. The more awareness you have about the subtle energies of your body, the more you can tune in and assess what's off balance and fix it.

The Least You Need to Know

- The five layers of your body are called the koshas. They are your physical, energetic, mental, intuitive, and bliss bodies.
- We are constantly picking up on signals like human radios.
- You are not the thoughts you think. They only exist in your mental layer.
- Underneath all of the koshas, people are all one; pure bliss.

CHAPTER 21

The Chakra System

The word *chakra* in Sanskrit means to wheel. In Ayurveda, this term relates to the wheels of energy throughout our bodies. In this chapter, we will discuss the seven chakras or energy centers in our bodies and what they relate to, giving you a deeper understanding of how imbalances in the mind connect to those in the body.

For example, if you constantly have a sore throat, that may be related to issues in your throat chakra. Headaches may be a sign of third-eye chakra imbalances. Menstrual issues could be related to sacral chakra problems. Let's explore the chakra-body connection.

In This Chapter

- The seven energy centers that run up and down your spine
- How your physical pain is related to your emotional
- What it means to be a soul having a human experience
- Tapping into your universal consciousness

What's a Chakra?

Of all the Sanskrit terms I've introduced you to in this book, you may be most familiar with *chakra* because it's often mentioned in yoga classes and spiritual texts. Chakras are energy centers that run along your spinal cord, from the top of your head down to the bottom of your tailbone. Each chakra is related to a particular energetic function, just like each kosha is (return to Chapter 20 if you need a refresher on koshas). In fact, the koshas and chakras are inherently related.

The Chakras

You have seven chakras: *muladhara* (root chakra), *svadhisthana* (sacral chakra), *manipura* (solar plexus chakra), *anahata* (heart chakra), *vishuddha* (throat chakra), *ajna* (third eye chakra), and *sahasrara* (crown chakra). Each is associated with a particular function and stored in a location in your body.

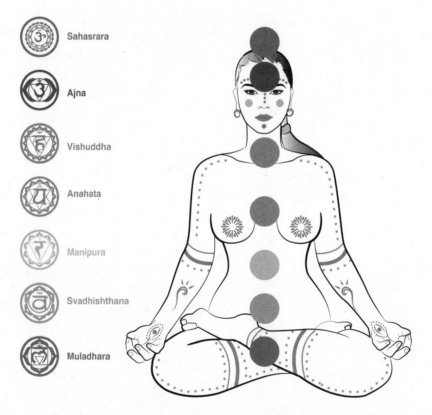

The chakras relate to various energy centers in the body and correspond to colors, symbols, elements, mantras and more.

The chakras, like the Doshas, can fall in and out of balance. In the following sections, I explain what the chakras are, the koshas and elements each is related to, the function of each, and symptoms of balance and imbalance.

To heal your chakras, you can use color, crystals, essential oils, and other types of natural therapies. I also share holistic ways you can bring your chakras back into balance, as well as mantras and affirmation for each.

Muladhara (Root Chakra)

The root chakra, *muladhara,* is the first of the seven chakras and is located at the base of your spine. Imagine your body is a tree; the root chakra is the roots. It is in charge of security, stability, and your most basic needs. This chakra is associated with the annamaya kosha, or the physical body, the earth element, and the color red.

Have you ever heard someone say you have to "keep your feet on the ground" or "stand your ground"? These ideas are associated with the root chakra, which provides strength and stability. It is primal in energy and controls your fight-or-flight response. The root chakra also relates to family and ancestry. You are spiritually connected to your ancestors, and any traumas they have gone through are stored in your root chakra.

Root chakra energy can make you feel communal and grounded as well as territorial and fear driven. When this chakra is in balance, you feel safe and self-assured. However, when it's out of balance, your fear patterns kick in, leaving you fearful, panicked, or uncertain. For example, when you lack a home and basic securities, your muladhara chakra falls out of balance.

I like to compare the chakras to Maslow's Hierarchy of Needs. The root chakra would be related to the first and most basic human need of physiological necessities: clean air, food, water, and sleep. Without these things, you won't be able to function. Root chakra imbalance is at the core of so many issues, in yourself and around the world, including war, famine, and violence.

> **WISDOM OF THE AGES**
>
> When you think of your root chakra, think survival, basic needs, security, family/tribe, and earthiness.

A person lacking root chakra energy may feel low in energy, ungrounded, insecure, anxious, or unstable. They may constantly be on a diet or suffer an eating disorder because they are disassociated from their body. Imbalances of the energetic chakras manifest as physical pain, and a person low in root chakra energy may feel pain in the hips, legs, or feet, the body parts associated with that chakra. They also may have disorders of the bones, a weak immune system, and/or constipation. All these imbalances relate to the Vata Dosha. Vata is extremely airy and lacks grounding, causing a root chakra imbalance.

A person with excess root chakra energy has too much energy in that center. They may feel angry, defensive, or competitive in nature. They also may be greedy, materialistic, or fixated on their routine and having a sense of security. These imbalances all relate to the Pitta Dosha, which can be very rigid and obsessed with achievements.

It is important to have a balanced root chakra so you have a strong sense of grounding without becoming inflexible.

Here are some tips to balance depleted root chakra energy:

- Connect with the earth's energy by spending time outdoors.
- Practice "earthing," walking in the soil with your bare feet to receive the negative ions from the earth.
- Eat more root vegetables and protein.
- Use the essential oil patchouli.
- Carry the crystals tourmaline, obsidian, jet, and hemamite.
- Practice saying the mantra "Vam."
- Repeat the affirmation "I am."

Svadhisthana (Sacral Chakra)

The second chakra, sacral, is located below your naval. It is your source of sensuality, sexuality, and creativity. The word *svadisthana* actually means "sweet." The "butterflies in your stomach" feeling comes from this passionate chakra. It allows us to connect with others in an intimate way and feel joy and pleasure. Relationships, movement, emotions, and the arts all arise from this sacred center. Svadisthana is associated with the pranamaya kosha, filling you with subtle creativity. It also relates to the fluid water element, in a constant state of flow.

When your sacral chakra is balanced, you are in touch with your emotions. You allow yourself to feel pleasure and can connect with others. Creativity channels through you, and you are tapped into your inner divine source. You may want to dance, move, and flow because you feel this feminine energy circulate through you.

> ### WISDOM OF THE AGES
>
> When you think of your sacral chakra, think relationships, pleasure, emotions, fertility, creativity, and wateriness.

When your sacral chakra is depleted, you are cut off from your emotions. You have trouble connecting with others and do not feel worthy of pleasure. You also may have reproductive issues or pain in your pelvic area. Fertility problems, sexual arousal disorder, skipped menstrual periods, lower back pain, shallow relationships, and communication problems with children are all signs of sacral chakra blockage. This relates to the Vata Dosha, which can be cold and flighty, afraid of depth and commitment.

When you have excess sacral energy, you may become overly emotional. Binge eating, fear of commitment, substance abuse, and mood swings are all associated with the sacral chakra. You might become addicted to an outside source such as sex, substances, or emotional abuse because you lack connection with your true self. This relates to the Kapha Dosha, which can become very emotional, as well as the Pitta, which can fall into addictions easily.

It is important to have a balanced sacral chakra so you can be in touch with your emotions without being driven by them.

Here are some tips to balance depleted sacral chakra energy:

- Express yourself artistically by drawing, writing, or painting.

- Move your body; practice yoga or dance.

- Feel your emotions, and don't be afraid of them.

- Seek counseling for sexual problems or addictions.

- Use the essential oil ylang.

- Swim in and spend time near the ocean.

Manipura (Solar Plexus Chakra)

The third chakra, solar plexus, is your power center. It decides who you are and what you are all about. It contains your ego self, your identity, and all aspects of your personality. Your self-esteem and willpower are part of the formidable *manipura* chakra. It is associated with the fire element and the color yellow. The manomaya kosha, your mental body, is associated with the solar plexus chakra because it contains your sense of self and mental prowess.

Your solar plexus chakra is located in your stomach, right below your rib cage. If you put your hands on that part of your body, you will feel heat. This is where your agni, digestive fire, lies. Your digestive organs, liver, pancreas, gallbladder, and upper intestines are all in this powerful area, as are your abdominal muscles. If you've ever heard someone say "He has no core," they're referring to this powerhouse chakra.

> **WISDOM OF THE AGES**
>
> When you think of your solar plexus chakra, think identity, power, energy, action, and fieriness.

When your solar plexus is depleted, you can easily lose yourself in others because you don't have a strong sense of who you are. This can lead to relationship issues, like the sacral chakra, but roots in your own lack of identity.

With a solar plexus depletion, you may have low self-esteem and willpower because you don't value yourself. You take on the victim mentality and blame others for your problems instead of owning up to them. Physically, this can lead to chronic fatigue, feeling cold all the time, stiff muscles, digestive issues, low appetite, back aches, and posture problems, all related to Vata Dosha because you lack that internal fire.

When you have excess solar plexus energy, you are obsessed with power and money. You become narcissistic and only see your own needs. You may have anger and control issues and always need to be the boss. You lack compassion for others and often become defensive and competitive. In the body, this manifests as hypertension, ulcers, stress, constant hunger, muscle spasms, and adrenal overload. Sounds like the Pitta Dosha, doesn't it?

It's important to keep your solar plexus chakra balanced so you have a strong sense of who you are without becoming overly attached to it.

Here are some tips to balance depleted solar plexus chakra energy:

- Practice core-strengthening exercises and aerobic exercise.

- Meditate twice a day, focusing on the fire in your core.

- Use the essential oil neroli.

- Carry yellow calcite and tigereye crystals.

- Spend 20 minutes in direct sunlight each day.

- Repeat the Sanskrit mantra "Ram."

- Say the affirmation "I can."

Anahata (Heart Chakra)

The heart wants what it wants, doesn't it? That's because the heart has its own intelligence, which often surpasses that of the mind. Your mind tells you what you are *supposed* to do based on previous experiences and expectations. Your heart only speaks the truth; it doesn't lie and deceive you the way your mind can. This is why it is so important to follow your heart.

The heart chakra, *anahata*, is located in the center of your chest and is actually associated with the color green, not red. It is associated with the vijnanamaya kosha, your intuitive body, and the air element.

> **WISDOM OF THE AGES**
>
> When you think of your heart chakra, think love, compassion, empathy, kindness, peace, and airiness.

The heart chakra is balanced when you are able to both give and receive love. You love others, but most importantly, you love yourself, too. You can love others only as much as you love yourself. If you do not love yourself first, you will be left depleted, without love to give. This will make you clingy and needy. You must treat yourself with the same compassion you give others.

When the heart chakra is balanced, you are overwhelmed with a feeling of love for everything. You may be sitting in your car and suddenly feel a wave of love, as I like to call it. You make your decisions from a heart-centered place and truly connect with others, seeing them for who they really are.

When this chakra is blocked, you give up on love. You may have been hurt in the past and have become fearful of opening your heart again. You're often closed off in your relationships and cold in your interactions. You may physically feel constricted in your chest area and suffer from heart attacks or breathing problems.

If you did not receive unconditional love as a child, you may have a blockage in your heart chakra. The true medicine is keeping your heart wide open, even when it's been abused or shattered. That's how you truly can become a vessel of love.

Here are some tips to balance depleted heart chakra energy:

- Practice self-care rituals like self-oil massage and dry brushing.
- Spend time with children and animals.
- Practice deep breathing with your hands on your heart.
- Do heart-opener yoga poses, such as backbends.
- Say the mantra "Yam" and the affirmation "I love."
- Carry a rose quartz or malachite.
- Use the essential oil chamomile.

Vishuddha (Throat Chakra)

The fifth chakra, *vishuddha,* is in your throat center and is in charge of communication. It's the energy center that not only houses your vocal cords but also propels you with the strength to always speak your truth and stand up for yourself. It allows you to be vocal, expressive, and collaborative. Writers, singers, and musicians often have open throat chakras. This chakra is associated with the color blue and the ether (space) element, which contains sound vibrations. It's linked to the vijnanamaya kosha because it is part of your intuitive body.

To have a strong throat chakra, it is just as important to be a good listener as it is to be a good speaker. Communication is a two-way street, yet a great orator is not necessarily a great communicator. Much of having an open throat chakra is being able to read between the lines. The true message lies not in the words but the meaning behind them. Those with strong communication skills can pick up on these subtle cues from others and are skilled conversationalists. They know how to speak to people and get their message across because they are extremely perceptive.

If you only speak but cannot listen, you may have excess third chakra (solar plexus) energy. If you only listen but cannot speak, you have excess heart chakra energy. Those with a good balance have open throat chakras.

> **WISDOM OF THE AGES**
>
> When you think of your throat chakra, think communication, truth, metaphorical thinking, and manifesting.

Those with balanced throat chakras are often musically gifted. They are able to pick up on vibrations, tones, melodies, and rhythms because they are in tune with sound vibration. They also may love to sing, even if they don't have a "good" voice, just because they like to utilize that chakra center.

Those with depleted throat chakra energy may have a hard time expressing how they feel. They have a fear of public speaking and a weak voice. They sometimes may lie to please others or take what others say too literally. This imbalance can manifest as physical issues such as a lump in the throat, sore throat, jaw tightness, neck stiffness, or strep throat. A depleted throat chakra often leads to hormonal issues due to hypothyroidism, which are all symptoms related to the Kapha Dosha.

Here are some tips for balancing depleted throat chakra energy:

- Sing your heart out!
- Practice mantras, especially the Sanskrit word "Ham."
- Repeat the affirmation "I express."
- Write every day.
- Get up and speak in front of others.
- Listen attentively.
- Use peppermint essential oil.
- Carry the crystals aquamarine and sodalite.

Ajna (Third Eye Chakra)

You see the physical world with your two eyes but you can tap into the unseen world with your third eye. Your third eye is your intuitive self. It's the knowing that something is going to happen right before it does. It's your inner psychic self who knows exactly what you need to do, even when your mind is telling you otherwise.

Your third eye chakra, *anja,* is essentially your sixth sense, able to perceive things based on subtle energies. If you've ever had a dream that later came true, that was your third eye chakra at work. It's related to all elements because it's pure light. When you practice visualizations, you are activating your ajna chakra. The color indigo is related to the third eye as well as the andamaya kosha, or bliss body.

> **WISDOM OF THE AGES**
>
> When you think of your third eye chakra, think intuition, inner wisdom, psychic vision, imagination, and dreams.

When your third eye is activated, you are an extremely perceptive being. You carry a deep, innate wisdom and can manifest your desires. You are highly intuitive and have very vivid dreams, which you tend to remember. Meditation comes naturally to you, and you are able to visualize to a great extent.

When your third eye is blocked, you wake up and can't remember a single one of your dreams. You make poor decisions and can't read people or foresee bad situations. You become materialistic and stuck in the rat race, without any thought of your significance in the world. You are out of touch with your imagination and turn to television for entertainment. You are overly stuck in the three-dimensional world—what you can see and touch—and lose touch with the magic of life you once saw as a child. This blockage can manifest as headaches, sinus infections, and nasal congestion, which are related to the overly grounded Kapha Dosha. You may even experience nearsightedness and night blindness.

Here are some tips to balance depleted third eye chakra energy:

- Write down your dreams as soon as you wake up.

- Practice meditation right after waking and again before sleeping.

- Do visualizations to activate your pineal gland.

- Use sandalwood essential oil.

- Express yourself creatively through art and music.

- Repeat the affirmation "Om."

- Say the mantra "I know."

- Carry the crystals labradorite, kyanite, and azurite lapis.

Sahasrara (Crown Chakra)

Now we've made it to the top of your head, your crown chakra. This chakra is above your physical body and connects you with the universal energy. The word *sahasrara* means "thousand-petaled" and is often symbolized by a lotus flower.

> **WISDOM OF THE AGES**
>
> The lotus flower represents the crown chakra because it is a beautiful white flower floating on the top of the water yet also has long roots that connect it to the ground below. Like the lotus flower, you must be rooted in the physical world, as muddy as it may be, to blossom into a beautiful flower above.

If you've ever had a moment of pure bliss, during which a warm sense of inner peace and gratitude overcame your entire being, that was your crown chakra being activated. Your crown is in charge of learning, spirituality, and your higher self. It is driven by education and always wants to find out more about who you are. Chances are, if you've picked up this book, your crown chakra is activated. The eternal quest for knowledge is part of the crown chakra.

Your crown chakra is your soul—who you are beneath your personality, thoughts, and physical body. It's the same you you've been all along and always will be. And deep down inside, everyone's souls are one. Everyone wants the same thing—love, connection, freedom, security, and purpose. When you truly realize people are all one and begin to live your life this way, you open your crown chakras.

When all seven chakras are open, your *kundalini* serpent energy is able to freely run up and down your spine, bringing you to enlightenment. Enlightenment is the realization that you are merely a soul having a human experience and were put on this planet for a greater purpose, to help others in whichever way the universe has gifted you. Some people are great writers, others are great caretakers, and others are strong leaders. Just like every person is born with a Doshic constitution, every person is born with a unique prevalence of their various chakras. This combination was set in place for you to fulfill your higher purpose, *dharma*.

> **WISDOM OF THE AGES**
>
> When you think of your crown chakra, think higher self/purpose, big-picture thinking, self-realization, enlightenment, and universal oneness.

With an open crown chakra, you are tuned in to the universal consciousness. What does universal consciousness even mean? If you've ever had a pet dog, you may notice him stretch in the classic "downward dog" pose when he gets up. No yoga teacher ever taught him how to stretch like that; he does it just because it's what his body innately needs. Similarly, even if you've never introduced him to another dog, he does "dog things," like circling around before he goes to sleep or digging in his bed area. He was never taught these things; this knowledge is the universal consciousness channeling through him.

The universal consciousness exists in all living beings. There have been many cases of animals stampeding before a big earthquake or birds migrating to a new part of the world before a hurricane. These animals didn't receive a memo bad stuff was coming; they were just tuned in to a source.

You are tapped into this universal energy, too. The only difference is you have a free-thinking mind that can override this innate wisdom and make you lose sight of your own wisdom. The universe is sending you messages all the time through your chakras. You just choose not to listen sometimes.

You are able to open your crown chakra when you realize that everything you see is a reflection of your internal state. You create your own realities based on your perceptions. You are not your name, your job, your personality, your family, or your story but rather a fleeting soul having a human experience. At the same time, you were put on this planet for a reason and have work to do. That work is not to pay bills, make a fortune, or have fame for the sake of it but instead to contribute something back to society in a meaningful way. Each person's meaning depends on his or her own unique skills received at birth from the stars.

To reach this level of self-actualization, you must be willing to do the work. Everyone has their own shadows, or repressed parts of themselves, to work on, such as jealousy, fear, or anger, which arise from their Doshas. You must be able to look at yourself without judgment, both your light and your darkness, to see who you truly are. Only then can you overcome your imbalances to step into your higher self.

When your crown chakra is blocked, you may feel out of touch with your own divinity. You may see yourself as worthless and become depressed. You may lack inspiration and purpose and go through the moves of life without truly living. Your body is there, but your soul is not.

Here are some tips to open the crown chakra:

- Keep learning about the world and yourself.

- Follow your curiosities.

- Make meditation a way of life.

- Be mindful of everything you do.

- Let go of unnecessary possessions and beliefs.

- Spend more time on your own and in nature.

- Practice a day in silence once a week.

- Study your ancestors.

- Stay in tune with your breath.

- Notice the beauty of life.

- Realize that everything happens for a reason and that there are no coincidences in life.

The following chart has everything you need to know about the chakras and koshas and all that they are related to, physically and mentally. Each line lists a specific chakra, it's related kosha, function, and associated physiology. I've further listed the symptoms of balance and imbalance of each and their associated color, essential oil, mantra, affirmation and crystal, showing you how to heal yourself holistically.

Balancing Chakras and Koshas

Chakra	Kosha	Function	Location in Body	Associated Physiology	When in Balance	When Imbalanced
Root	Annamaya	Survival	Base of spine	Hips, sacrum, legs, feet, lower intestines, joints, bones, coccygeal nerve plexus	Stable, grounded	Fear, primal instincts
Sacral	Pranamaya	Sensuality	Below naval	Sex organs, lower back, abdomen, bladder, pelvis, sacral nerve plexus	Good relationships	Unable to be intimate
Solar plexus	Manomaya	Identity	Base of rib cage	Stomach, gastrointestinal tract, adrenals, organs, middle back, solar nerve plexus	Strong sense of self	Anger, power-hungry
Heart	Vijnanamaya	Love	Center of chest	Thymus gland, heart, lungs, breasts, shoulders, cardiac nerve plexus	Able to give and receive love	Closed off to connections
Throat	Vijnanamaya	Communication	Throat	Thyroid, throat, trachea, neck, pharyngeal nerve plexus	Expressive and outspoken	Unable to speak the truth, thyroid and sinus issues
Third eye	Anandamaya	Intuition	Third eye	Pineal and pituitary glands, carotid nerve plexus	Deep awareness and understanding	Out of touch with higher self, materialistic
Crown	Anandamaya	Enlightenment	Top of head	Brain, nervous system, pituitary and pineal glands, cerebral cortex	Self-actualization, bliss	Lack of belief, skeptic

Color	Element	Essential Oil	Mantra	Affirmation	Natural Therapy	Crystal
Red	Earth	Patchouli	"Lam"	"I am"	Connecting to the earth	Obsidian, jet, hematite
Orange	Water	Ylang	"Vam"	"I feel"	Sexual expression	Garnet, ruby
Yellow	Fire	Neroli	"Ram"	"I can"	Sun-bathing	Yellow calcite, tigereye
Green	Air	Chamomile	"Yam"	"I love"	Self-care	Rose quartz, malachite
Blue	Ether	Peppermint	"Ham"	"I express"	Singing and chanting	Aquamarine, sodalite
Indigo	All	Sandalwood	"Om"	"I know"	Creative expression, dreaming	Labradorite, kyanite, azurite lapis

The Least You Need to Know

- You have seven chakras, or energy centers, that lie along your body's energy pathway and correspond to a specific area of your physical, emotional, and spiritual well-being.

- The seven chakras are the root, sacral, solar plexus, heart, third eye, and crown chakra.

- The first three chakras are more physical, and the second three are more intuitive. The crown chakra is above the body.

- The root chakra is in charge of survival. The sacral chakra relates to sexuality. The solar plexus chakra holds your power.

- The heart chakra gives you the ability to give and receive love. The throat chakra allows you to communicate impeccably. The third eye chakra connects you with your intuition. The crown chakra is your relationship with the higher source, universal consciousness.

- When your chakras are balanced, you experience enlightenment.

PART 6

Ayurvedic Healing

In this last part of the book, you learn how to apply this ancient healing wisdom to your modern life and reap the benefits of panchakarma, the ultimate detox treatment. I also provide some home remedies for everything from digestive disorders, to skin conditions, to everyday illnesses, empowering you to become your very own healer.

Panchakarma

Panchakarma is one of the most well-known parts about Ayurveda. It is a five-step, total mind-body rejuvenation experience complete with herbalized oil massages, steam therapies, enemas, a cleansing *kitchari* diet, and other toxin-purifying practices.

Panchakarma helps eliminate toxins from your body, rebalance your Doshas, heal countless ailments, and give you a renewed sense of clarity and inner peace. It is an immersive experience that requires the participant to stay in a Panchakarma facility for between 3 and 21 days for the full treatment. The average Panchakarma is 5 days. However, it isn't like a normal spa holiday with poolside massages and green juices. It is a mind-body experience that will remove toxins from every part of your body.

In This Chapter

- Panchakarma: the ultimate detoxification treatment
- Why people flock to India for Panchakarma
- The most cleansing diet to consume to remove toxins
- What the Panchakarma experience entails

The Panchakarma Experience

I remember my first Panchakarma experience in India. I was lying on a wooden massage table as two women rubbed a thick layer of pungent herbalized sesame oil into every square inch of my body—a scent I'll never forget.

As I lay there in a state of bliss, I suddenly jumped up with a nose full of oil. I didn't realize at the time, but the ladies had squirted oil up my nose as part of nasya, or nasal irrigation.

The day continued with ghee—lots of ghee. This clarified butter made its way into almost every facet of the experience, from the cupfuls I drank on an empty stomach every morning to my undereyes to enemas.

Not only were the treatments extremely detoxifying, but also no mental stimulation was permitted so we could really be present in the experience. Technology was not allowed, and the center where I was, overlooking the Indian Ocean, did not even have electricity in the bamboo huts we stayed in. We were in bed by sunset and up to the sounds of the chickens at sunrise, ready for our oil-filled treatments.

They say Panchakarma is not for the faint of heart, and I have to agree. It pushes your mind, body, and spirit to a level you may have never experienced before, purging out the old and stale from your colon, stomach, and mind. However, you walk away from it a renewed person, open to the possibilities of life.

About Panchakarma

Panchakarma means "five therapies" in Sanskrit. These five therapies are the most detoxifying treatments in Ayurvedic medicine, cleansing all channels of your body and removing toxins that may later cause illness. It basically takes an imbalanced body, lathers it up with oil, and brings it back into balance.

The five traditional therapies of Panchakarma are *basti* (herbalized oil enemas), *nasya* (nasal irrigation), *vamana* (therapeutic vomiting), *virechana* (purging), and *raktamokshana* (bloodletting). However, most of these treatments are no longer practiced today and have been replaced with milder, more relaxing treatments such as oil massages and gentle therapies.

Panchakarma is internationally known for its ability to cure almost any ailment, from eczema to diabetes to heart disease. It's one of the most purifying things you can do for yourself and causes you to become so much more aware of the toxins you are holding onto, physically as well as emotionally.

Panchakarma is recommended not only to treat ailments but also to prevent diseases caused by seasonal changes. As the seasons shift, toxins accumulate in your system. This is why Panchakarma is recommended every seasonal shift to keep your Doshas in balance.

Panchakarma is serious work, even though you aren't physically doing anything. In fact, for many, that's what makes it so difficult. Your body is releasing years of stored toxins, and even though you're sitting still the entire day, you end up exhausted by the time your daily treatments are over.

> **WISDOM OF THE AGES**
>
> The purpose of Panchakarma is *sodhana*, purification. According to the Charaka Samhita, Ayurveda's oldest text, if a disease is treated with sodhana, it does not reoccur. Panchakarma is the ultimate way to heal and rebalance the body.

The Benefits of Panchakarma

Panchakarma's many benefits include the following:

- Cleared toxins from your entire system
- Balanced Doshas
- Healed digestive system
- Enhanced immunity
- Decreased stress
- Antiaging
- Improved skin luster
- Weight loss (if overweight)
- Deep relaxation
- Meditative outlook in life
- Enhanced mindfulness

Pre-Panchakarma

Before Panchakarma, it's recommended that you cleanse your body in a process called oleation. You're encouraged to only eat kitchari, lentils and rice in healing spices, or at least simple, vegetarian cooked meals for at least a week before your Panchakarma experience. You also should take ghee or castor oil to help cleanse your bowels and loosen toxins before beginning the program. You also should refrain from eating meat, excess travel, anger, stress, and other unbalancing foods and experiences.

A Typical Day of Panchakarma

Each person will have his or her own Panchakarma experience because it is personalized for the individual, but in this section, I want to give you an idea of what a day in Panchakarma might look like.

The first thing you do is meet with the Ayurvedic doctor who will check your tongue; assess your pulse; and have you fill out forms about your digestive patterns, cravings, health goals, medical history, mental characteristics, skin, metabolism, dreams, and much more. It's a very detailed questionnaire that assesses all facets of your body and disposition.

With that information, the doctor will prescribe your Panchakarma experience unique to your specific needs.

A typical day may look like this:

Wake up with sunrise and practice yoga and meditation.

Drink a cup of ghee with specific herbs for your imbalances. (The ghee helps the herbs better absorb in your system.)

Begin your first treatment of the day, such as an oil massage or enema.

Spend time in the steam bath to release toxins.

Eat a detoxifying lunch of kitchari.

Walk around in nature, or sit and meditate.

Undergo another treatment, such as shirodhara, third eye therapy.

Consume a light dinner of more kitchari or cooked vegetables and rice.

Read, meditate, and head to bed to rest up for another healing day.

The Panchakarma Diet

What makes Panchakarma so effective is the diet you follow while on the program. You're on a strict diet of just kitchari, which is basmati rice and lentils slow cooked in medicinal spices and herbs.

You cannot drink alcohol, coffee, or anything besides tea. You also cannot eat salads or smoothies because they are too cooling and light for the system. Meat, bread, and sugar are also off the list because they are too heating and heavy for the system.

Your diet is completely sattvic, pure and evoking positivity, to evoke ojas, well-being. If you continue eating sandwiches, pizza, and processed foods, the Panchakarma therapies will have no effect. Cleansing begins within, and the kitchari diet is a crucial part of the Panchakarma experience.

In the process of Panchakarma, you become extremely aware of your own food addictions, such as something sweet after meals, a crunchy snack, or piece of chocolate in the afternoon. Everything is soupy, well cooked, and simple. Some Panchakarma centers offer an assortment of Ayurvedic foods and even fruit, while more traditional ones only serve kitchari.

Ghee, or clarified butter, is considered liquid gold in Ayurveda and is the superstar of the Panchakarma experience, making its way into almost every treatment and meal.

Herb-infused oils are used abundantly as well, both in cooking and therapies. These oils help release deep-seated toxins from your system for total purification.

Panchakarma Therapies

Most Panchakarma facilities today focus on the relaxing and nourishing treatments, such as massages, rather than the more intensive therapies, such as purgation. Let's look at some of the more popular Panchakarma therapies.

Shirodhara (Third Eye Therapy)

Shirodhara is one of the most recognized treatments in Ayurveda because of its uniqueness. In this divine treatment, a steady flow of warm oil is poured onto your third eye center, on your forehead between your eyebrows, to awaken your intuitive self. The word *shiro* means "head," and *dhara* means "continuous flow of liquid."

Benefits of shirodhara include the following:

- Activated third eye center

- Headache and migraine relief

- Reduced anxiety, stress, and depression

- Relaxed nervous system

- Balanced excess Vata

- Improved sleep

- Heightened senses

- Softened wrinkles

- Improved cognition

Abhyanga (Oil Massage)

I spoke about abhyanga self-oil massage in Chapter 11, but this treatment also can be performed by a professional Ayurvedic massage therapist or two for even deeper benefits. During this massage, the practitioner(s) warm the oil, infuse it with herbs specialized for your Dosha, and apply it along your body's energy channels using a specific method to increase your Prana life force.

This massage stimulates your lymphatic drainage, removes toxins, and reduces stress. Your head, stomach, feet, hands, legs, back, neck, and shoulders are all massaged during a session that usually lasts 2 hours.

Afterward, you sit in a steam bath to help remove stored cellular waste. You are not permitted to shower afterward so the oil can sit on your skin for at least 24 hours.

Many facilities have two-person massages during which two practitioners massage your body at the same time for double the bliss.

Benefits of abhyanga include the following:

- Released toxins

- Unblocked energy channels

- Enhanced Prana and breathing

- Relaxed sense of self

- Improved digestion

- Released muscular tension

- Decreased muscle stiffness

- Rejuvenated mind, body, and spirit

Karna Purana (Ear Therapy)

Karna purana, or ear therapy, is recommended for those with hearing or ear problems. In this treatment, your neck and head are massaged with oil, followed by a warm ear steaming. Your ears are then massaged and covered with a hot towel. Herbalized oil is poured into your ears until your ear cavity is full of oil, and you sit up to allow the oil to completely enter your ear crevice. This treatment is especially recommended for those who spend a lot of time on their phones or in loud areas.

Benefits of karna purana include the following:

- Improved hearing

- Reduced ear wax, mucus, and yeast

- Cleared sinuses

- Reduced ear ringing

- Decreased jaw and facial tension

Nabhi Basti (Digestion Therapy)

Nabhi basti is an interesting treatment performed to improve digestion and release stored emotions. In this treatment, your abdomen is gently massaged with herbalized oil to remove toxins and enhance digestion and elimination. Then, a dam is created out of dough around your belly button. The circle is filled with warm herbalized oil, and you relax with the oil pooled on you for 30 minutes. This treatment is great for those with low digestive fires, irritable bowel syndrome, or other gastrointestinal issues.

Benefits of nahbi basti include the following:

- Improved digestion

- Released deep-seated emotions

- Enhanced elimination

- Decreased constipation, bloating, gas, and indigestion

Netra Basti (Eye Rejuvenation Therapy)

Netra basti is a treatment especially for your eyes. It's similar to nabhi basti, in that a dam is created out of dough and filled with oil. This time, the dam is around your eye socket. You close your eyes, the dough dam is placed above your closed eye, and it's filled with warm herbalized ghee. (If some ghee gets in your eyes, it won't hurt, and it's actually recommended to enhance your vision.) You rest with the oil above your eyes for 30 minutes.

Benefits of netra basti include the following:

- Improved vision

- Rested, rejuvenated eyes

- Decreased dry eye and eye tension

- Softened wrinkles and crow's-feet

- Decreased dark circles

Hrid Basti (Heart Opening Therapy)

In *hrid basti,* the heart is the center. Oil is massaged over your heart to open your heart chakra and increase love, warmness, strength, and nourishment. This therapy is effective for treating respiratory issues, heart disease, stress, and asthma as well. All you need is love!

Benefits of hrid basti include the following:

- Increased feelings of love, union, connection, and joy

- Opened heart chakra

- Decreased stress

- Improved breathing

- Strengthened heart muscle

- Decreased cardiac risk

Udvartanam (Dry Powder Massage)

Udvartanam is one of the only Ayurvedic treatments performed without oil. In this therapy, dry herbal powder is rubbed on your body to stimulate your lymphs and balance your Kapha Dosha. The treatment helps break down fatty deposits, treating obesity and cellulite. It increases circulation, stimulates metabolism, and removes toxins, all while exfoliating your skin.

Benefits of udvartanam include the following:

- Weight loss

- Detoxification

- Softened skin

- Lymphatic drainage

- Increased blood flow

Shiro Abhyanga (Head Massage)

Shiro abhyanga is all about the head. In this massage, your marma (energy) points are gently massaged to relieve tension, clear your mind, and even promote hair growth. Sesame oil infused with *brahmi,* a specific herb for hair health, is massaged into your head, leaving you in a state of bliss.

Benefits of shiro abhyanga include the following:

- Reduced headaches

- Improved hair quality and growth

- Enhanced sleep

- Cleared mind

- Increased mental peace and alertness

- Decreased depression, anxiety, and anger

At-Home Panchakarma

Anyone can benefit from a detox because your body is constantly creating toxins. Even if you lived in a perfect world with all organic food, clean air, and no stress, your body still would produce toxins. So it's important to cleanse regularly.

> **WISDOM OF THE AGES**
>
> Do you have a thick layer of coating on your tongue? Are you tired throughout the day, especially after meals? Do you have body aches and pains? Do you have uncontrollable cravings? Is your mind foggy? Do you have bad-smelling breath, body odor, or flatulence? Do you have constipation or diarrhea? These are all signs you need to detox.

However, detoxification does not necessarily have to be at a Panchakarma facility. You can perform many Ayurvedic detoxification therapies yourself, at home, such as abhyanga self-oil massage, nasya nasal irrigation, a cleansing kitchari diet, herbal laxatives, an oil enema, a technology detox, daily yoga, meditation, and sleeping and waking early.

Here's an example of what your at-home Panchakarma day might look like:

Wake up at sunrise.

Tongue scrape and oil pull.

Drink hot water with ginger, cumin, cinnamon, coriander, and cardamom.

Practice meditation and yoga.

Eat a cleansing breakfast of kitchari.

Massage your body with warm sesame oil.

Take a hot shower, and rest in the steam.

Read or relax while drinking more tea.

Eat a cleansing lunch of kitchari.

Massage oil into your scalp, naval, or heart.

Rest or take a walk in nature.

Meditate and practice gentle yoga.

Dry brush your body, and apply more oil.

Drink tea with triphala (a cleansing Ayurvedic herb)

Get to sleep by sunset.

Now here's a great kitchari recipe you can try.

Healing Tridoshic Kitchari

Kitchari is the ultimate healing recipe for all Doshas. It's warming, easy to digest, and extremely healing for the agni. It promotes ojas, good health, and longevity and is totally sattvic, enhancing positivity, clarity, and joy. It's full of prana life force and gives your overused digestive system a chance to rest so your body can heal. Kitchari is simple, delicious, and well balanced with the six tastes. It makes the perfect Panchakarma meal, but you can enjoy it anytime you feel like you need a detox.

3 TB. sesame oil, coconut oil, or ghee

1 tsp. mustard seeds

1 tsp. cumin seeds

1 cinnamon stick

6 cardamom pods

1 (2-in.) piece ginger, peeled and grated (2 TB.)

$1/2$ tsp. turmeric

2 pinches asafetida (optional)

$1/2$ tsp. sea salt

1 cup basmati rice, soaked overnight, drained, and rinsed

1 cup yellow split mung beans, soaked overnight, drained, and rinsed

1 or 2 pieces kombu (optional)

8 cups water

Juice of $1/2$ lime (optional)

1. In a large pot over medium heat, heat sesame oil. Add mustard seeds, and cook, shaking the pot occasionally, until you hear a popping sound. (This means mustard seeds are activated.)

2. Add cumin seeds, cinnamon stick, cardamom pods, ginger, turmeric, asafetida (if using), and sea salt, and cook, stirring, for 30 seconds.

3. Add basmati rice, mung beans, and kombu (if using), and cook, stirring, for about 1 minute to meld flavors.

4. Add water, and bring to a boil. Stir, reduce heat to simmer, cover, and cook for about 1 hour or until water is mostly absorbed and mixture has a creamy consistency similar to risotto. (You could add the mixture to a rice cooker at this point and cook for 30 minutes.)

5. Remove from heat, add lime juice (if using), and serve.

WISDOM OF THE AGES

If beans are hard for you to digest, I recommend adding a bit of kombu, a sea vegetable that coats the beans with digestive enzymes. This will decrease your flatulence and make the nutrients even more accessible to your body.

The Least You Need to Know

- Panchakarma is the ultimate detoxification treatment in Ayurveda.
- This 3- to 21-day experience clears toxins; balances the Doshas; enhances digestion; decreases stress; and rejuvenates the body, mind, and spirit.
- Eating a cleansing and simple kitchari diet of easy-to-digest spiced lentils and basmati rice further promotes detoxification.
- The Panchakarma experience involves various oil-filled treatments, such as third eye therapy and digestive, ear, and head massage.

CHAPTER 23

Ayurvedic Home Remedies

You've learned so much up to this point, and I hope you've been practicing some Ayurvedic self-care. Now let's look at how you can help heal your friends and family with tried-and-true methods from Ayurvedic wisdom.

Ayurveda was the first system ever to see plants as medicine, and modern Herbology actually derives from Ayurveda. When Ayurveda went underground during the British rule of India, it became a "kitchen medicine," meaning people used the herbs and spices in their kitchens to heal. For this reason, Ayurveda contains lots of home remedies, teas, and tonics to treat everything from everyday colds to constipation.

Keep in mind these remedies do not replace going to your doctor, and you should always consult your physician before beginning any health-care regimen changes.

In This Chapter

- Using ingredients in your kitchen to cure many common ailments
- Healing digestion with the help of herbs
- Pampering your skin with plants
- Balancing your hormones through holistic health

Digestive Disorders

A healthy gut is the key to a healthy life. People in the Western world often experience digestive disorders due to processed foods; eating on the go; and consuming too much salt, sugar, and fat (and not the good kind). The remedies in this chapter help heal a number of digestive disorders so you can eat without pain.

Remember, prevention is key. The best way to treat a digestive disorder is to prevent it from coming along in the first place. Look out for foods that give you an upset stomach by keeping a food log or journal.

> **WISDOM OF THE AGES**
>
> You might be sensitive to certain ingredients and have no idea. The most common culprits are corn, peanuts, soy, dairy, eggs, gluten, wheat, nuts, shellfish, sugar, and artificial sweeteners. Remove all these from your diet, and see if your symptoms get better. If not, look at other specific ingredients you may be eating that cause problems. For example, I had no idea I was sensitive to pineapple and was eating it regularly. I didn't have an immediate reaction, but it caused digestive discomfort. Not all food sensitivities are immediate. Some can manifest hours or even days later.

Until you figure out the cause of your digestive discomfort, here are some home remedies you can use in the meantime to heal your body with natural ingredients. Some of these ingredients you may already have, some are for sale in your local market, and others you'll have to order from an Ayurvedic herb company. (I listed some sources for herbs in Appendix B.)

Stomachache

Stomachaches are quite common. However, not all stomachaches are the same. They can be the result of a host of different causes, from improper digestion to constipation and even appendicitis.

To treat a stomachache, you must first know its cause. If it's a sharp pain, see your physician.

If it's a normal stomachache caused by something you ate, try the following remedies:

- Boil 4 cups water. Add 1 tablespoon fennel seeds, 1 teaspoon cumin seeds, and ½ tablespoon fresh grated ginger. Steep for at least 20 minutes. Drink warm.

- Combine 2 tablespoons lemon or lime juice, 2 tablespoons ginger juice or grated ginger, and 1 cup water. Drink as needed.

- Chew on fennel seeds after your meals.

Constipation

Constipation can be caused by numerous imbalances. Primarily, it's caused by excess Vata, which leads to colon dryness. Secondarily, it can be caused by a sedentary lifestyle, which is actually Kapha related. Thirdly, it can be caused by too much meat and acidic foods in the diet, which is Pitta related.

Constipation also can occur when you're dehydrated or don't consume enough fibrous foods, such as vegetables and fruit. Mentally, constipation can occur when you place too much mental strain on yourself, which actually can cause physical strain on your body. It can result from your inability to let go and can actually stem from childhood traumas. Take a look at your lifestyle, see what could be the cause of your constipation, and treat accordingly.

Here are some remedies for treating constipation:

- For a quick fix to constipation, boil 1 cup water and add 1 tablespoon flaxseeds and 1 teaspoon cumin. Steep for 10 minutes, and drink the contents of the cup, including the seeds. You should have a bowel movement by the morning.

- Psyllium husk is very effective at treating constipation. Add 1 tablespoon to a glass of water and drink, or add it to meals for extra fiber intake.

- Triphala is my favorite herb for preventing constipation. Unlike laxatives, it does not force your muscles to loosen up to create a bowel movement and is safe for everyday use. Triphala heals digestion and naturally helps clean out the colon. I recommend taking take a capsule at morning and at night, especially for dry Vata types.

- If your constipation is caused by mental strain, practice meditation. Allow your mind to come into stillness, and let go of lingering negative thoughts, tensions, and insecurities. Come to peace with yourself and the present moment. Focus on surrender and letting go.

WISDOM OF THE AGES

Keep a journal, and note when you feel constipated and what's going on in your life at that moment. You may notice it's when you have a stressful day at work or you get into a fight with your spouse. When you're aware of the cause, you can take preventative measures to avoid the problem.

Gas and Bloating

It's normal to experience gas. In fact, it's estimated that the average person passes gas 14 times a day. Ayurveda doesn't recommend holding in gas because that can cause the air to circulate in your system. So find a private place and discretely pass your gas.

Gas is caused by excess air in your system, which is attributed to the Vata Dosha. When you eat dry, cold, or rough foods, such as raw foods, fibrous vegetables, and popcorn, gas accumulates in your system. If you don't have a strong digestive fire, the food will build up, undigested, and cause fermentation. The odorous gas is a result of this putrification.

Similarly, bloating is caused by excess air in your stomach that distends your belly. It's also caused by a weak digestive fire, leaving your food to sit in your stomach undigested. This can lead to excess bad bacteria growing in your colon, leading to candida, a yeast that attributes to sugar cravings, yeast infections, and digestive disorders.

If you are experiencing gas or bloating, try these remedies:

- Boil 4 cups water, and add 2 tablespoon cumin seeds. Steep for at least 10 minutes. Drink warm throughout the day. (This is both preventative and acute.)

- In 1 cup room temperature water, combine 2 tablespoons lemon juice, 1 teaspoon apple cider vinegar, and ½ teaspoon baking soda. Drink before and after meals to alkalize your body and neutralize gas.

- Chew on fennel seeds after meals. Adding fennel seeds to your meals also promotes digestion. Fennel tea is effective as well.

- Chew on fresh gingerroot with salt after meals. Simply peel ginger and sprinkle on a small amount of sea salt, then chew it and swallow it's juices. Ginger tea is effective, too.

- Avoid raw foods, salads, and carbonated drinks. Favor warm, cooked, easily digestible meals like blended vegetable soup and mung beans.

- Avoid cold water and drinks, such as iced tea, smoothies, iced coffee, and ice water. Drink only warm or hot beverages.

Heartburn

Heartburn is caused by a Pitta imbalance, attributing to excess acid in the stomach. Pitta is fire energy in charge of all transformation in the body, so when your system contains excess fire, you become overly acidic. This acidity actually leaves your stomach and trickles up your esophagus, which is why you experience heartburn. Many heartburn sufferers actually have low stomach acid because the acid has all moved up. It's important to neutralize your pH and remove all acidic, Pitta-aggravating foods from your diet.

Here are some ideas for combatting heartburn:

- Don't eat meat. Meat is very acid forming and can cause hyperacidity in your body, which begins with heartburn but can lead to many diseases.

- Eliminate Pitta-aggravating foods such as garlic, onions, pickles, fermented foods, citrus fruits, and coffee.

- Drink 1 cup aloe vera juice in the morning on an empty stomach. Drink more after your meals to sooth your body. You can take aloe capsules if you prefer.

- On an empty stomach or at least one hour before meals, in 1 cup room temperature water, combine 2 tablespoons lemon juice, 1 teaspoon apple cider vinegar, and ½ teaspoon baking soda. Drink 1 to 3 times a day. Not only does this help gas and bloating, but it also neutralizes acidity.

- Eat mindfully and slowly. Oftentimes heartburn is the result of indigestion brought on by eating too quickly. Be present during your meals, chew each bite until it dissolves from your mouth, and wait 20 minutes before taking second portions. (It takes 20 minutes for your body to know that it's full.)

Indigestion

Indigestion is very common today, thanks to our habit of eating on the go and choosing processed foods, among other digestively unhealthy reasons. Indigestion manifests as pain or cramps after meals. It results from your digestive fire not being able to break down your food.

Heavy, dense foods, such as fried and oily foods, meat, cheese, and bread, tend to cause indigestion. However, if your digestive fire is weak, just about anything can trigger it. It's important to eliminate all heavy foods from your diet to allow your digestive fire to rebuild.

The way you eat can result in indigestion, too. If you emotionally eat, stuffing your body without any consideration of how much food you're actually ingesting, your digestive system will have to work harder, causing indigestion. Improper food combining is another huge cause of indigestion (more on that in Chapter 17).

If you suffer from indigestion, try the following remedies:

- Drink ginger tea, especially before and after meals, to kindle your digestive fire and make you better able to break down food. I recommend grating fresh ginger in hot water and steeping it for at least 20 minutes.

- Take trikatu, an Ayurvedic herb made of ginger, black pepper, and Indian long pepper.

- Do not eat until your body is truly hungry. Drink herbal tea between meals to give your body a chance to digest.

- Massage your stomach lightly to promote digestion.

- Take a walk after a heavy meal to jump-start your metabolism. You'll feel much lighter after some activity.

- Add spices to your meals. Cumin, fennel seeds, and mustard seeds make your foods easier to digest.

- Drink hot water with cinnamon instead of having a sugary dessert. It will satisfy your sweet tooth while helping kindle your digestive fire.

Diarrhea

It's normal to experience diarrhea at some point in your life. Diarrhea happens when your body rejects something you ate. It might have contained a bacteria or other pathogen your body is protecting you from. It also happens when the Pitta Dosha is aggravated and your digestive system goes into overdrive to evacuate everything.

Diarrhea means your digestive system is too weak to break down the food, resulting in loose stools. It's often triggered by Pitta foods, such as spicy meals or fermented foods. To rebuild your digestive fire, eat a simpler, sattvic diet.

Try these remedies, too:

- Take shatavari, an Ayurvedic herb, to combat chronic loose stools.

- When your bowels are loose, drink ½ cup room temperature water mixed with ½ cup plain unsweetened yogurt and 1 pinch sea salt.

- Eat a very simple diet of rice and cooked vegetables until the diarrhea has subsided. Avoid any spiced foods, meat, garlic, onions, tomatoes, or anything else that will imbalance Pitta. Oatmeal is also fine.

- Drink raw coconut water to battle dehydration and replenish potassium levels.

- Eat ripe bananas to help bind the stool and replenish potassium levels.

- Boil 2 cups hot water, and add 1 teaspoon fennel seeds. Steep for at least 10 minutes, and drink.

AYURVEDIC ALERT

Diarrhea is the body's defense mechanism against a potentially harmful virus or bacteria. Diarrhea also results from inflammation in the colon, related to the Pitta Dosha. If you are having diarrhea for more than 2 or 3 days, please consult a doctor because you could be losing vital fluids.

Intestinal Parasites

Parasites are actually more common than you'd believe and can come from the foods you eat. The most common parasites found in the human intestines are roundworms, pinworms, whipworms, threadworms, diardia, hookworms, and tapeworms.

If you experience an increased, insatiable appetite; digestive discomfort; bloating; illness; or other symptoms, get checked for parasites. If you have traveled to a tropical country, you are more at risk of having parasites. The best way to know for sure is to get a stool test conducted by a medical professional.

If you are positive for parasites, try the following treatments:

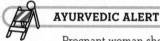 **AYURVEDIC ALERT**

Pregnant woman should not follow any of these suggestions. Consult your doctor instead.

- Take neem, also known as Indian lilac. This herb not only kills parasites but also aids the removal of the toxicity they leave behind. Take a neem supplement, or buy dried leaves to make tea.

- Ayurvedic herbs amalaki, bibhitaki, haritaki, pippali, kutaja bark, and vidanga all combat parasites. Tablets that combine these ingredients to combat intestinal worms are available.

- Consume more bitter and pungent foods, like leafy greens—spinach, kale, collards, mustard, and dandelion greens—and garlic. These have properties to kill the parasites.

- Add coconut oil, which is antiparasitic and helps expel parasites, to your diet while killing parasites to promote their evacuation.

- Pumpkin seeds can be effective at getting rid of intestinal worms and are actually recommended by the University of Maryland Medical Center. They contain a compound called cucurbitacin that paralyzes parasites and prevents them from latching on to the intestinal walls. The best way to get the benefits is to boil them in water, steep for 30 minutes, and drink the "tea" throughout the day.

- Make hot tea of cloves to destroy parasitic eggs and kill worms within the body. Boil 1 cup water and add 1 ground clove. Steep for 5 minutes, and drink throughout the day.

- Add turmeric to everything. Not only is it great for digestion, it also kills parasites. Turmeric is heat-activated and best in cooked foods and warm beverages, especially with black pepper.

> **WISDOM OF THE AGES**
>
> Ayurveda believes that intestinal parasites are caused by a weak digestive fire, creating an ideal situation for parasites to thrive. Parasites are more likely to affect Vatas and Kaphas because they have weaker digestive fires.

Candida Overgrowth

Candida albicans is a naturally occurring intestinal inhabitant we all have in our guts. However, when our digestive fire is not hot enough, the candida yeast overgrows and spreads throughout our intestines, overrunning our good gut bacteria. It then enters our blood stream, causing candida overgrowth. Yeast infections, thrush, digestive issues, sugar cravings, cystic acne, and lethargy are all signs of candida overgrowth. If you notice that you crave sugar daily, regularly suffer from yeast infections, experience oral thrush, or have chronic infections throughout your body, you likely suffer from candida overgrowth. You can test for candida overgrowth with a saliva or blood test.

It's estimated up to 80 percent of the population has an overgrowth of this candida due to our sugar-centric diet.

If you experience the earlier symptoms and tested positive for Candida, try the following suggestions:

- Remove all sugar from your diet, including bread; pasta; rice; honey; maple syrup; processed foods; and even all fruits except berries, coconut, and avocados. Any type of sugar can feed candida, including fructose. Switch to natural sugar alternatives, such as monk fruit sweetener, organic liquid stevia, or birchwood xylitol.

- Add more bitter and pungent foods to your diet, particularly garlic, asparagus, dandelion greens, collard greens, kale, and spinach.

- Increase the cruciferous vegetables in your diet. Broccoli, cauliflower, and kale help scrape out yeast overgrowth in your gut.

- Take neem. This bitter herb helps kill excess bad bacteria to rebalance a healthy gut flora.

- Take amalaki, bibhitaki, haritaki, pippali, kutaja bark, and vidanga, available in tablets from Ayurvedic herbal supplement companies.

- Incorporate coconut oil, which is antifungal and helps expel bad bacteria from your system, to your diet while cleansing from candida.

- Add psyllium husk powder to your diet to aid the removal of candida.

> **WISDOM OF THE AGES**
>
> Most of the guidelines for cleansing from Candida are the same as those for intestinal worms because they are both considered ama, an internal toxin. But there are minor differences. Candida comes from an overgrowth of yeast that's already inside of you, while parasites are caused from an external source.

Skin Problems

Ayurveda is very effective at treating skin blemishes. External beauty begins within, and Ayurveda has both internal and external remedies for healing the skin so you can radiate with vibrant health.

Acne

Acne is one of the most embarrassing kinds of blemishes, especially if you suffer from it as an adult. Ayurveda states that acne comes from excess Pitta. Heat rises, so if you have too much fire in your system, it has nowhere to escape and comes through your pores, turning into pimples. Pittas naturally have oily faces and are most sensitive to toxicity, making them high risk for breakouts. The more toxic their diet, the worse their acne. Acne also can be caused by stress, hormonal imbalance, premenstrual syndrome (PMS), air pollution, improper digestion, and candida overgrowth.

To heal acne, follow these guidelines:

- Remove all oily foods from your diet, including fried foods, tempuras, chips, red meat, nuts, stir-fries, and oil-rich soups. Excess oil in the diet will show up on your skin.

- Avoid spicy foods, fermented foods, nightshade vegetables, garlic, onions, salt, and citrus fruits, which all aggravate Pitta. Follow a more sattvic diet of basmati rice; legumes; and cooling vegetables like asparagus, cucumbers, and leafy greens.

- Boil 4 cups water, and add 1 teaspoon cardamom, 1 teaspoon saffron, and 1 teaspoon fennel seeds. Steep for at least 10 minutes, and drink warm throughout the day.

- Drink cucumber water throughout the day, and rub cucumber on your skin to cool down redness and inflammation. To make cucumber water, add several slices of cucumber to room temperature water.

- Cleanse your skin with rose water nightly.

- Make a mask with 1 cup plain organic yogurt, 1 teaspoon turmeric, and 1 teaspoon raw honey. Apply to your face, let sit for 15 minutes, and wash off with warm water. Do not leave on for longer than recommended because turmeric can turn your skin slightly orange. This mask helps clear toxicity from your pores and brightens your complexion.

Dry Skin

Opposite of oily skin, dry skin is still a problem. No matter what you do, your skin feels parched and tight. Although you might be grateful you don't have breakouts caused by oily skin, you might run into another problem. Because overly dry skin can cause wrinkles and fine lines, your skin lacks hydration. Dry skin is caused by excess Vata. Vata is a cold, dry energy that leaves your skin parched.

Moisturizers, lotions, and creams are not the answer because they don't address the root cause of the dryness: internal dehydration. Follow a Vata-pacifying diet so your skin regains its suppleness.

Oils also are used in Ayurvedic tradition because they don't exhaust the sebaceous glands like moisturizers do, which can cause more dryness. Oils penetrate the pores more deeply than creams and don't contain the chemicals store-bought lotions do. You never should put something on your skin you wouldn't eat because both enter your blood stream.

If you have dry skin, try the following remedies:

- Avoid dry, rough foods, including raw vegetables, crackers, granola, and popcorn. Favor soft, oil-rich foods like vegetables cooked in coconut oil, soups, mashed sweet potatoes, and curries.

- Do not use soaps on your skin. These only further dry it out. Instead, use oils to cleanse your skin and remove your makeup.

- Use oils to moisturize as well. Sesame oil is most recommended for Vatas and can be applied to your entire body daily.

- Apply a facemask of ½ mashed avocado and 1 teaspoon raw honey. Leave it on your face for 15 minutes, and wash off with warm water. These ingredients will leave your skin feeling hydrated and replenished, so repeat as needed.

Damaged Skin

Skin damage has many culprits, including the sun, stress, pollution, and age, all of which can leave your skin looking dull, flaky, hyperpigmented, swollen, wrinkly, and red.

If your skin is damaged from the natural wear and tear of life, try the following remedies:

- Consume more antioxidant-rich foods like berries, pomegranates, and amla (Indian gooseberries).

- Avoid coffee, alcohol, cigarettes, and secondhand smoke.

- Drink warm water throughout the day to hydrate your skin.

- Consume more leafy greens and citrus fruits, both of which are high in vitamin C.

- Make rejuvenating hydrating mask by combining ½ mashed banana, 1 tablespoon ground oatmeal, and 1 tablespoon milk. Place on your skin for 15 minutes, and wash off with warm water.

- Smash tomatoes and place them on your face for 15 minutes and then wash off with warm water.

WISDOM OF THE AGES

Bananas are considered nature's Botox because they contain potassium, which heals blemishes, as well as antioxidants that help eradicate the free radicals that cause aging. Tomatoes are very high in vitamin A, which regenerates damaged skin. They also are high in vitamin B, which promotes cell renewal, and vitamin C, which stimulates cellular metabolism.

Dark Undereye Circles

Dark circles make you look haggard and exhausted, no matter how much you slept. They can be caused by two reasons: dark pigmentation under the eyes, which many Indian women have, and thin skin around the eyes, which many Caucasian women have. Dark circles are caused by lack of sleep, dehydration, alcohol, smoking, an unhealthy diet, stress, dryness, and aging, too. However, there is a fix.

To heal dark undereye circles, try the following:

- Crush 1 tomato in a small bowl, and add ½ teaspoon lemon juice and a pinch of turmeric. Apply to your dark circles, being careful not to get the mixture in your eyes because it may burn. After 15 minutes, wash off with warm water.

- Juice 1 cucumber and 1 potato. Dip cotton pads in the juice, and place them on your eyes. Relax for 15 minutes with the pads on your eyes and then wash your face with warm water.

Common Illnesses

Ayurvedic remedies can be used to cure almost any everyday ailment! The following sections offer remedies for some common illnesses.

Headaches

Sometimes, headaches can be just awful to deal with. Ayurveda classifies headaches into the three Dosha types: Vata, Pitta, and Kapha. Vata headaches typically occur at the back of your head or on the left side and are caused by anxiety or overthinking. Pitta headaches are in the temple area and caused by anger or too much heat. Kapha headaches are in the frontal and nasal areas and are caused by sinus congestion and poor circulation.

Here are some remedies to help combat headaches:

- To reduce Vata headaches, make a paste of sesame oil and nutmeg and rub it into your forehead. Leave it on for at least 30 minutes and then take a hot shower. Follow a warming, grounding diet, and try an enema.

- To reduce Pitta headaches, make a paste of sandalwood powder and water and rub it into your forehead. Leave it on for at least 30 minutes. Stay away from bright lights and the hot sun. Take 2 tablespoons aloe vera several times a day, and eat something naturally sweet.

- To reduce Kapha headaches, make a paste of ginger powder and water and apply it to your forehead. Leave it on for at least 30 minutes. Rinse your nostrils with salt water, and practice yoga.

Migraines

Migraines are more severe than headaches and are often caused by a Pitta imbalance. Excess Pitta can constrict the blood vessels around your brain, causing pressure on your nerves.

If you're battling a migraine, these things might help:

- Avoid bright light and sunlight.

- Follow a cooling, Pitta-pacifying diet.

- Take the Ayurvedic herbs shatavari and brahmi.

- Take slow, deep breaths, focusing on the exhale to remove heat from the body.

Colds and Flus

We all get sick sometimes, but as we become more balanced, the occurrences will be less often and severe. What used to be several days home sick can turn into a few measly sniffles, thanks to these Ayurvedic remedies:

- Boil 1 cup water. Add 1 tablespoon grated ginger, 1 teaspoon cinnamon, and 1 teaspoon cardamom. Steep for 10 minutes, and drink.

- Eliminate Kapha-unbalancing foods from your diet.

- Put 3 to 5 drops of ghee in your nostrils in the morning and at night.

- Take the Ayurvedic herb amlakai, which is very high in vitamin C.

Fevers

Fevers occur when there's too much toxicity, ama, in your system, making your body unable to fight off an infection. To heal a fever, it's important to cool your body from within.

Ayurveda recommends not consuming much if you have a fever to give your digestive system a time to rest so your body can heal itself.

Try these teas, too. I recommend sipping them throughout the day, every 30 minutes to stay hydrated.

- To relieve feeling hot, drink mint tea made with hot water and several mint leaves.

- To kill infection, drink holy basil and tulsi tea.

- To rebuild digestive strength, drink an herbal remedy of hot water with 1 teaspoon cumin, 1 teaspoon coriander, and 1 teaspoon fennel seeds. Drink as needed.

Women's Health

Ladies, Ayurvedic remedies can help keep your flows in sync and your bodies healthy!

PMS and Cramping

If you have any type of pain around your period, something is out of balance. Ayurveda classifies three Doshic types of menstrual difficulties and suggests specific treatment for each:

- For Vatas, pain occurs before the onset of your period, often with cramps, bloating, lower stomach and back pain, insomnia, and scanty blood. To treat, take ashwaghanda and rub castor oil on your belly.

- For Pittas, congestion, inflammation, tender breasts, hot flashes, irritability, and heavy flow can be problems. To treat, take shatavari and rub coconut oil on your belly.

- For Kaphas, pain occurs in the latter part of the cycle, often with water retention, heaviness, exhaustion, cravings, and lethargy. To treat, take trikatu and rub mustard and castor oil on your belly.

- All Doshas should chew on 1 teaspoon cumin seeds followed by a drink of 1 tablespoon aloe vera juice, drink hot water with cinnamon, and consume fresh raspberries with raspberry leaf tea.

Irregular or Missed Menstrual Cycles

Irregular or missed periods can be caused by a Vata imbalance, leading to low hormonal levels. When a woman is underweight, on a low-fat diet, overexercising, or under stress, she may skip her period. It's important to restabilize and ground your body so it can get back into the flow of things.

> **AYURVEDIC ALERT**
>
> Missed periods for more than 3 months, called amenorrhea, can contribute to bone density issues later in life, such as osteoporosis, so it's essential to address the underlying cause before it turns into a lifelong issue.

Here are some suggestions you might try:

- Follow a Vata-pacifying diet with warm cooked foods, healthy fats, and sesame oil.

- Consume sesame seed milk made of ground sesame seeds mixed in water.

- Take shatavari, an Ayurvedic herb that improves female sexual health.

Urinary Tract Infections

If you've ever felt a burning sensation when you've had to pee, that's likely a urinary tract infection (UTI). Have no fear—Ayurveda has a cure for that:

- Take the Ayurvedic herbs shilajit and amlaki.

- Make a tea with 1 cup hot water and 1 teaspoon coriander seeds. Steep for at least 10 minutes, and drink three times a day.

- Avoid Pitta-aggravating foods like spices, chile peppers, coffee, and alcohol.

- Drink unsweetened raw cranberry juice.

The Least You Need to Know

- The ancient Ayurvedic texts contains thousands of herbal remedies for virtually any ailment under the sun.
- Ayurveda looks at the root cause of an issue and addresses it from the source.
- As a kitchen science, Ayurveda believes in healing the body through the one thing we do three times a day—eat. Each meal should contain medicinal herbs and spices to bring you back into balance.
- Let plants be thy medicine and thy medicine be plants; side effects not included.

Glossary

abhyanga The ancient Ayurvedic practice of massaging the skin with oil to hydrate the body from within. It enhances muscle tone, detoxification, and relaxation.

agni Your internal fire, in charge of digestion, nutrient assimilation, metabolism, and creation of bodily tissues. When agni is healthy, you are able to easily digest both foods and emotions, making you physically and mentally sound. When agni is too much or too little, you begin suffering from digestive, health, and emotional issues.

Ayurveda The world's oldest health system. It originated in India 5,000 years ago with the goal of achieving mind-body balance. It contains medical, spiritual, psychological, and philosophical components, all focused on promoting lifelong wellness.

chakras The energy centers along your spinal cord, from the top of your head down to the bottom of your tailbone. Each chakra is related to a particular energetic function: root chakra (muladhara), sacral chakra (svadhisthana), solar plexus chakra (manipura), heart chakra (anahata), throat chakra (vishuddha), third eye chakra (agna), and crown chakra (sahasrara).

dhatus The seven bodily tissues: plasma, bones, muscles, fat, nervous system, and reproductive system.

dinacharya Your daily practice, such as brushing your teeth, washing your face, scraping your tongue, oiling your body, meditating, and eating breakfast. The term means "to be close to the day" because balance is found when you work with the rhythms of nature.

Dosha The Ayurvedic term for "energy" used to describe all people, foods, and things. The three Doshas are Vata (air and ether), Pitta (fire and water), and Kapha (earth and water). *See also* Kapha; Pitta; Vata.

dry brushing The Ayurvedic practice of gently scraping the body with a dry loofa brush to remove toxins and dead skin cells and stimulate the lymphatic system.

Kapha   The Ayurvedic Dosha comprised of earth and water elements, governing your bone density and all structure within your body. When Kapha is out of balance, you experience heaviness, fatigue, water retention, depression, and other related issues. *See also* Pitta; Vata.

koshas   The five layers surrounding your physical body that comprise your whole being. These five layers are your physical body (annamaya), energy body (pranamaya), mental body (manomaya), intuitive body (vijnanamaya), and blissful body (anandamaya).

nasya   The Ayurvedic practice of administering oil up your nose to heal allergies, improve breathing, relieve headaches, and even improve quality of voice.

neti   The Ayurvedic practice of rinsing out your nostrils with salt water to treat congestion and improve breathing.

ojas   The subtle essence related to health and well-being. It makes you peaceful and patient. *See also* prana; tejas.

panchakarma   An ancient Ayurvedic fivefold detoxification and rejuvenation method involving herbalized oil massages, steam therapies, enemas, a cleansing *kitchari* diet, and other toxin-purifying practices.

Pitta   The Ayurvedic Dosha comprised of fire and water elements, governing your stomach and all transformation within your body. When Pitta is out of balance, you experience heartburn, overheating, anger, impatience, and other related issues. *See also* Kapha; Vata.

Prakriti   The Doshic constitution you were born with, determined at the moment of conception. For example, you may have been born primarily Kapha, secondarily Vata, and lastly Pitta. *See also* Vikruti.

prana   The subtle essence related to vital life force and breath. It makes you flexible and creative. *See also* ojas; tejas.

rajas   The universal quality representing movement, passion, and energy. It fills you with power, but excess can lead to aggression. Stimulants, nonvegetarian foods, and pungent tastes are considered rajasic.

rasa   The Ayurvedic term for taste. The six tastes are sweet (madhura), sour (amla), salty (lavana), bitter (tikta), pungent (katu), and astringent (kashaya).

sattva   The universal quality representing purity, clarity, and potential energy. It illuminates you with knowledge, wisdom, compassion, and enlightenment. Fresh vegetables, fruit, certain grains, and easily digestible meals are considered sattvic.

self-actualization   The achievement of your full potential through creativity, independence, spontaneity, and a grasp of the real world.

tamas   The universal quality representing inertia, inactivity, and lethargy. Tamasic foods include processed and frozen meals, refined sugar and carbs, meat, alcohol, onions, and garlic.

tejas   The subtle essence related to radiance and glow. It makes you intelligent and courageous. *See also* ojas; prana.

Upavedas   The secondary Vedic teachings that go into four technical subjects: the arts (Gandharvaveda), warfare (Dhanurveda), health (Ayurveda), and architecture (Sthapartaveda).

Vata   The Ayurvedic Dosha comprised of air and ether elements, regulating your nervous system and all movements within your body. When Vata is out of balance, you experience constipation, bloating, anxiety, irregular periods, and other related issues. *See also* Kapha; Pitta.

Vikruti   The Doshic constitution you have today due to your diet, environment, lifestyle, and other factors. For example, you may eat many cold foods and live in a cold place, making your Vikruti Vata. *See also* Prakriti.

Resources

I want to thank you for taking the time to read this book, creating a ripple effect of healing on this planet. I hope I have shown you how easy it is to apply Ayurvedic wisdom in your life and you use this book as a tool to heal your friends, family and the world. Healing the planet begins with healing yourself and I am so proud of you for beginning the journey. Thank you for making me part of it.

I am so overwhelmed with gratitude for the positive feedback I have gotten since this book has been released in August 2017. I never could have imagined within one day, this book would become the #1 Best-Seller in Ayurveda. I wrote this book as the exact healing tool I wish I had on my journey and I am so honored that my modern approach to Ayurveda has resonated with so many of you across the planet. Many of you have shared on social media using this book in your yoga teacher-trainings, wellness events, health-coaching programs, moon circles and other gatherings and I am overjoyed to see that this book has taken a life of its own. May the Vedas live on, through me and through you.

Sahara Rose Ketabi

If you enjoyed reading this book and would like to learn more about my modern approach to ancient Ayurveda, I invite you to check out my website SaharaRoseKetabi.com where I offer an interactive mind-body type quiz that leads into a free 3-day Eat Right For Your Mind-Body Type mini-course. Unlike any other Ayurvedic quiz, I separate the results between the mind and body's Dosha because I have found that people often totally relate to one physically and another mentally. I also break down each Dosha by percentage, giving you a detailed overview of your unique characteristics today.

If you'd like to take it a step further, I offer a 12-week *Eat Right for Your Mind-Body Type* online guided program in which I teach you how to apply this ancient Ayurvedic wisdom to your life, step by step, in a modern, approachable way. I have updated and simplified this complex healing system, the way I did in this book, so even the busiest person with no experience in the kitchen can reap the benefits of Ayurveda. Side effects may include improved digestion, increased energy, radiant skin, effortless weight loss, eliminated cravings, and a deep feeling of mind-body balance. Don't say I didn't warn you!

I also share weekly blog posts, recipes, quizzes, and free gifts on my website. You also can log on to find out where I'm teaching workshops in the Los Angeles area or retreats around the world, covering topics from sacred self-care to healing your relationship with food. I'm currently working on a cookbook inspired by the goddesses from around the world as well as a natural skincare line, so stay tuned for that as well by subscribing to my email list

Bring me with you on your commute! I host of the Highest Self Podcast, which focuses on the next step of wellness: using this radiant health so you can go out there, share your gifts and fulfill your purpose on this planet. I discuss how your Dosha is connected to your Dharma (life's purpose), discovering your soul's archetype, understanding your past lives and more. The Highest Self Podcast available on iTunes, Soundcloud and Stitcher.

Hungry for more? I am currently working on my next book, Eat Feel Fresh, which is a modern Ayurvedic cookbook using plant-based ingredients from around the world so stay tuned for that by subscribing to my mailing list!

Let's bring the sacred back to social media. Be sure to connect with me on Instagram, Facebook, YouTube and Twitter @IAmSaharaRose for daily mind-body-spirit inspiration and to stay updated on my offerings. I can't wait to connect with you there.

Other Ayurvedic Books

As mentioned earlier, many Ayurvedic books have been written. Here are a few others you might find useful.

Chopra, Deepak, MD. *Perfect Health*. New York, New York: Three Rivers Press, 2001.

Lad, Vasant, BAMS, MASc. *Ayurveda: The Science of Self-Healing*. Twin Lakes, Wisconsin: Lotus Press, 1985.

————. *The Complete Book of Ayurvedic Home Remedies*. New York, New York: Harmony Books, 1999.

Lutzker, Talya. *The Ayurvedic Vegan Kitchen*. Summertown, Tennessee: Book Publishing Company, 2012.

O'Donnell, Kate. *The Everyday Ayurveda Cookbook*. Boulder, Colorado: Shambhala Publications, 2015.

Svoboda, Robert, Dr. *Prakriti*. Twin Lakes, Wisconsin: Lotus Press, 1998.

Yarema, Thomas, MD, Daniel Rhoda, DAS, and Johnny Brannigan. *Eat Taste Heal*. Kapaa, Hawaii: Five Elements Press, 2006.

Ayurvedic Herbal Supplement Companies

There are plenty of beneficial Ayurvedic herbs to take that balance the body and mind. It's important to buy your herbs from a supplier that sources their herbs consciously and organically. Here are some of my favorite companies.

Ayush Herbs
ayush.com

Banyan Botanicals
banyanbotanicals.com

Organic India
us.organicindia.com

Sun Potion
Sunpotion.com

VPK by Maharishi Ayurveda
mapi.com

Ayurvedic Panchakarma Centers

Ayurvedic Healing
Santa Cruz, California
ayurvedichealing.net

The Ayurvedic Spa
Nevada City, California
be-vital.com

Chopra Center
Carlsbad, California
chopra.com

Life Spa
Boulder, Colorado
lifespa.com

The Raj
Fairfield, Iowa
theraj.com

Index